where he met his wife Hitty. Shortly after that he went into general practice at Kew Gardens in Surrey, where his son Patrick was born in 1952. While practising there he became medical correspondent of the *News Chronicle* and later of the *Daily Mail*. In 1965 he gave up general practice to go into hospital psychiatry. He gained the Diploma in Psychological Medicine in 1967 and was then appointed to the permanent psychiatric staff at Park Prewett Hospital, Basingstoke.

Since a trip to America in 1958 to promote his best-seller *Eat Fat and Grow Slim*, he has been working on the allergy approach to mental illness, which was demonstrated to him by doctors in Chicago. Lately he has set up an out-patient clinic for patients with food and chemical allergy at Basingstoke District Hospital and has published several papers on the subject in the medical journals. An account of his work and results in this field, *Not All in the Mind*, is published in Pan.

He now runs the Chemical Victims Club in Basingstoke, and is supported in his research work by a grant from the Wessex Regional Health Authority.

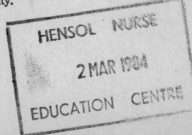

Also by Richard Mackarness
in Pan Books

Not All in the Mind

RICHARD MACKARNESS
MB BS DPM

Chemical Victims

PAN ORIGINAL
Pan Books London and Sydney

First published 1980 by Pan Books Ltd
Cavaye Place, London SW10 9PG
Second Printing 1980
© Richard Mackarness 1980
ISBN 0 330 25937 7
Made and printed in Great Britain by
C. Nicholls & Company Ltd, The Philips Park Press, Manchester

to William J. Rea MD FACS
thoracic and cardiovascular surgeon,
Director of the Brookhaven Environmental Control Unit,
Dallas, Texas,
for his help and encouragement with this book

The most powerful antigen known to man is a new idea.
Wilfred Trotter (1877–1939)

Consulting Surgeon to University College Hospital, London;
Honorary Surgeon to the King (1928–32)

Contents

Acknowledgements   viii

Foreword by Dr Kenneth Vickery MD FFCM DPH   xi

Author's note   xv

1 A background to clinical ecology   1

2 The discovery of allergy   21

3 A case of chemical allergy?   43

4 Chemical adulteration of food   53

5 My own and other cases   68

6 Drugs as toxins   90

7 Gas and indoor air pollution   104

8 Extending the ecological approach   115

9 Chemical victims of industry   133

10 Questions and answers   142

Epilogue   156

Appendices and References   161

Index   191

Acknowledgements

I wish to acknowledge the help I have had from a number of people in the writing of this book and in the practice of clinical ecology.

At Basingstoke District Hospital:

Dr John Fowler, Consultant Physician; Dr Hugh Platt, Clinical Tutor; Jeannette Bealer and Maxine Freeman in the Postgraduate Centre; and Dilys Smith and her staff in the Medical Library there.

Sister Price, Sister Thorn and Staff Nurse Sheila Steyning in the Outpatient Department and the nursing staff on 'E' floor (Medical), 'G' floor (Children), and on the wards in the Psychiatric Division.

Mr Fennell and his staff in the Pharmacy, the Catering Department and the two dieticians, Rosanne Spencer-Smith and Joan Benham-Crosswell.

Still in Hampshire, I want to thank Dr William Mckee and Dr Robert Rowe at the Wessex Regional Health Authority and Professor Jack Howell, Dean of Southampton University Medical School, for their support for research I have been doing.

Moving further afield – Dr Théron Randolph, Dr Bill Rea, Dr Lawrence Dickey, Dr Robert Collier, Dr Doris Rapp, Dr Joe Miller and Dr Murray Carroll of the Society for Clinical Ecology in America, for teaching me so much that has gone into this book.

The members of the Chemical Victims Club, particularly 'Loretta' and 'David' who allowed me to use their stories in this book.

So many colleagues inside and outside medicine have helped me, that it would be impossible to name them all. I must, however, thank Dr Kenneth Barlow, Dr Barbara Latto, Dr Andrew Strigner and Mrs Herta Larive, fellow members of the committee of the McCarrison Society, for all their encouragement. Also Margery Hall, Joy Warren and the other committee members of the charity Sanity who have supported my work on the nutritional and biochemical factors in mental illness.

Sonny Mehta and Kyle Cathie at Pan Books have been good to me and so have Peter Grose and his secretary, Linda Van, at Curtis Brown, the literary agency which took me on when I was struggling to get my previous book, *Not All in the Mind*, published.

I apologize to anyone I have omitted to mention and say thank you to my secretary, Jean Green, for her hard work and good temper, to my wife Hitty and my son, Patrick, for making me such a nice home to come back to after work.

R.M. 1979.

PERMISSIONS

The author and publishers wish to thank the following for their kind permission to quote extracts:

Dr Théron G. Randolph and his publishers, Charles C. Thomas of Springfield, Illinois, USA, for *Human Ecology and Susceptibility to the Chemical Environment*.

Leslie Kenton and the proprietors of *Harpers & Queen* for *The Chemistry of Consciousness*.

Nursing Times for the article on 'Allergy to Food and Chemicals' by Sue Todd and Richard Mackarness.

Dr E. Binkley and Dr Murray Carroll for their papers given at the Advanced Seminar in Clinical Ecology, San Francisco, 1977.

Dr Doris Rapp and her publishers, Sovereign Books, for extracts from *Allergies and the Hyperactive Child*.

Beatrice Trum Hunter and her publishers, Allen & Unwin, for *The Mirage of Safety*.

Dr Irving Selikoff for his paper on the Michigan disaster, given at the Advanced Seminar in Clinical Ecology, Key Biscayne, Florida, in 1978.

Foreword
by

Kenneth Vickery MD FFCM DPH
Consultant Community Physician, Chairman of Council, The
Royal Institute of Public Health and Hygiene

*I am pleased to have enlisted Dr Kenneth Vickery's interest in my
researches. In the course of some thirty years in preventive medicine
he has consistently highlighted environmental factors in public health,
particularly the over-consumption of refined carbohydrate and the
need for dietary fibre. This, and his work on the hazards of old age,
has placed him ahead of his time in community medicine. I do not
think he will regret his early recognition of the potential of
clinical ecology, which is a logical extension of his pioneering work.*

R.M.

There are few more frustrating experiences in life than to feel
persistently unwell, to be suffering from very real and even disabling symptoms, to be given a routine series of investigations by
general practitioner and specialist, only to be assured that nothing
organically wrong has been found and, therefore, to be expected
to feel better and forget about it.

This last quarter of the twentieth century will undoubtedly
attract descriptive biological captions. It can already be called
the age of epidemiology: the study of health and disease in
populations having achieved at least as high a place in the
hierarchy of inquiry as the elusive results of contrived double-
blind trials. This is also undoubtedly the age of the environment,
which the more enlightened will like to call the age of ecology,
with emerging appreciation that the health of man can only be
adequately studied in the context of his living surroundings
inclusive of the living soil from which he is made and to which
his physical remains return.

For many a weary sufferer, however – and it is a function of community medicine to pursue such matters – these times must surely be felt as the age of psychosomatic presumption or the age of psychogenic dismissal, or simply the age of n.a.d. (nothing abnormal discovered).

It is the sequel to n.a.d. which can be the really devastating part for many, with the apologetic 'I don't for a moment think you are mentally ill or that you are imagining your symptoms, but I do think that if they persist a psychiatrist may be the only answer', which being loosely translated can mean 'Pull yourself together or you may find yourself on the couch in the bin.'

Undoubtedly, some n.a.d. patients may be in need of the psychiatrist's ministrations but it has now fallen to a perceptive psychiatrist to be one of the first medical men in Britain to establish that certain troublesome symptoms of many of his patients may indeed have an essentially physical rather than psychiatric cause. To perceive in fact that they may be victims of new twentieth-century environmental insults arising from contact with sensitizing substances in the food, water or in the air – in short they are victims of masked allergy to chemicals.

Notwithstanding tremendous advances in the elimination of the killer infectious diseases, in the expectation of life from birth and in the reduction of the drudgery of everyday living, can we really be surprised that there is a price to be paid in this age which has spawned simultaneously a population explosion and a technological revolution? An age which has seen more dramatic change in food and in the chemical environment in the last 150 years than in the previous fifteen million. The fact is, and it is a principle of Darwin from which few have differed, man and all living species are possessed of remarkable powers of adaptation to a changing environment. Such adaptation is, however, geared to the climatic pace of nature's changes. The powers of adaptation are not yet fitted to the pace of this generation's dramatic man-made environmental changes. The parents of many alive today were born before the chug of the first internal combustion engine and before the first steel roller mill began the baleful process of the mass production of denatured flour.

So it comes about that Richard Mackarness, whose observations on food allergy described in *Not All in the Mind* are being increasingly recognized in the medical press and clinical practice, now casts the net wider to consider the allergic implications of a host of chemical pollutants ranging from car exhaust fumes, domestic gas, aerosol propellants, insecticides, herbicides, detergents and therapeutic drugs, right down to synthetic underwear. He presents convincing evidence of widespread hypersensitivity and maladaptation to these as well as previously described foods and food contaminants. Such is the foundation for the new, but already respectable, study of clinical ecology.

A consideration of the case histories given, with relief achieved after years of unsuspected allergy, is bound to raise the question that this whole subject may be a paradise for hypochondriacs. May not this book be avidly seized upon by the many patients who are convinced their doctors don't understand them? Will they not use such a book to pester the life out of their GPs, demanding to be referred to specialists and departments of clinical ecology which do not yet sufficiently exist?

Possibly so, but also there could well be the likelihood that some of the supposed hypochondriacs may be helped. Moreover, the potential of diagnosis for many others, which rings so true in these pages, surely justifies the publicizing of this credible new speciality. Nor should there be any real danger in the short-term self-diagnostic elimination procedures including the Stone Age diet, provided no long-term exotic dietaries or regimes are adopted without medical sanction. The evidence of these pages adds further justification to the efforts of those, hitherto often so glibly ridiculed, who bother to grow, market or buy organically nurtured and minimally processed foods and who seek to live apart from the grosser pollutions of mankind.

There is only so much the individual can do to avoid chemical pollutants or to become desensitized. General protection is dependent upon central and local government policies such as the strict car exhaust emission requirements in Japan and the USA. Food and agriculture mass-production objectives, however, present a finely balanced problem in the face of demands of hungry populations. Whether we like it or not, the present world-wide shortfall in oil supply, having regard to the rising toll of petrochemical sensitivities not to mention malignancies, could well be a blessing in disguise provided alternative non-polluting sources of energy can be exploited. Electricity continues to be the least environmentally harmful form of energy. A strong case can already be made for converting natural gas, coal and oil into electricity rather than the hazardous distribution and local burning of these pollutant fossil fuels. The capital and revenue costs of such policies must be weighed against the costs in resources, life and limb of the incessant digging up of the streets to sustain a now ageing gaspipe network and of bulk distribution of fuels. With abundant, cheap electricity available, the way would be open to conversion of water into hydrogen and oxygen thus providing, in one operation, unlimited non-polluting fuel *and* a means of offsetting the menace of too much carbon dioxide in the atmosphere.

We may well conclude that the caption of the times with the most serious implications for man's continued life on earth is 'the age of pollution'. Certainly the comfortable equation *mens sana in corpore sano* is now incomplete without the addition of a further dimension which is *in vicinia sana* (in a healthy environment).

AUTHOR'S NOTE

Although this book is called *Chemical Victims*, it is partly about food allergy, because foods are chemicals in the strict sense of the word. Food allergy cannot be separated from chemical allergy in a book on the victims of the chemical environment, because almost everything we eat now contains chemical additives and contaminants. A more accurate, though far too abstruse, title for this book would have been 'Clinical Ecology' – a comparatively new branch of medicine which is concerned with maladaptive or allergic reactions to the food we eat, the water we drink and the air we breathe. Professor William Rea, to whom I have dedicated this book and who is himself a 'chemical victim', once said he was 'allergic to the twentieth century'. As pollution of our environment grows, so more and more of us are becoming ill in mysterious ways attributable to an inability to adapt and stay healthy in our increasingly contaminated chemical environment. A complete re-appraisal of medical and public health priorities is called for if we are to avoid going the way of the dodo and the dinosaurs.

PUBLISHER'S NOTE

Explanatory footnotes appear at the bottom of the page; references indicated by numbers in the text can be found at the back of the book on pages 187–90.

ONE

A background to clinical ecology

The crowd parted to let an ambulance man through to the girl who lay unconscious in the road. She had been walking back to her office after lunch, in the busy Hampshire town of Basingstoke. She was not a casualty in a road traffic accident, though she might easily have become one. Eventually, she was to be one of the first patients I treated for allergy to chemicals; in her case motor car exhaust fumes and related hydrocarbons. That was in 1975. Today she is fit and working in a new job and is one of the leading members of the Chemical Victims Club which I help to run for people like her: a sort of Allergics Anonymous. I will call her Loretta and she is typical of the growing membership of the club. Of her illness, she wrote:

I was in the Metropolitan Police Force and I left to marry Arthur who was a Police Constable. I was ill as a WPC and I used to faint 'on the beat'. At the time of my referral to you, I was a secretary in Basingstoke ... very clean office ... lots of sprays and polish. At that time married to Arthur for a year, I was managing to hold down a job – just – in spite of the fainting which came on without warning, and attacks of this terrible skin rash. I used to have to go to bed at 6 p.m. every working night, taking half a child's dose of antihistamine: Piriton tablets.

It sent me instantly to sleep for twelve hours and made me dopy next day, but it controlled my urticaria to some extent so that I was able to keep my job. But it did nothing for the fainting, which was very alarming. Every job I'd had since leaving school (five or six in all) I had to leave through ill-health and embarrassment about sick leave. Except the Police Force, which I left to get married.

My GP referred me to Dr Fowler, who told me, 'Giant urticaria has never been known to last longer than ten years...' Five years down, five to go! When I asked to be referred to you, having read an article about you in a magazine, he refused at first, but later agreed.

When Loretta used to collapse on the pavement, people would rush to her aid and rather to her subsequent annoyance start pummelling her chest and trying to give her the kiss of life. She would regain consciousness within a short time, with or without these unwelcome ministrations from keen and usually male passers-by and then, within twenty minutes or so, would break out in an itchy rash all over her body.

Various doctors whom she had consulted over the years had been baffled and in 1975, soon after she had come to live in Basingstoke, Dr John Fowler, one of the Consultant Physicians at the District Hospital, rather reluctantly sent her to me. His reluctance was not so much that he did not know what I was doing – he did – but because I am a psychiatrist and like most down-to-earth physicians he has a deep suspicion of psychiatrists. Here is the discharge report which I sent to him and to Loretta's GP after I had treated her on a ward in the Psychiatric Division:

Reason for Referral
Repeated attacks of giant urticaria accompanied by fainting.

Brief History
She had been a policewoman and more recently a secretary, but had to give up work because of her illness which had not resolved with antihistamines.

Mental State on Admission
Good. No rash when first seen.

Investigations
Full blood count, electrolytes, chest X-ray and urinalysis: all negative.

Treatment and Progress in Hospital

She was put through our usual routine for suspected allergy patients, i.e. was fasted for five days on nothing but bottled spring water (Schweppes Malvern) and then given challenges with watery extracts of the various foods she had been eating, dropped under her tongue. A number of these brought back her fainting but not the urticarial rash: white sugar, milk, sardines, cornflour, cabbage, Ryvita, molasses and banana.

Most of the foods tested produced no reactions, so that on discharge she had a wide choice of foods from which to build a compatible diet.

During her fast, accidental exposure to a 'Freshaire' aerosol spray being used by a ward orderly in a bathroom was followed by fainting and a rapid return of her urticaria.

Thereafter, she was challenged on separate days with single inhalations of all the sprays which she had been using regularly at home, and which she had been forbidden to use in hospital. All, including her perfume and deodorant aerosols, caused fainting and massive return of her urticaria. A paper bagful of motor car exhaust fumes had the same devastating effect.

On Wednesday 2 April she was again shown at the weekly Postgraduate Clinical Meeting at the Basingstoke District General Hospital (the physicians had shown her previously as a problem patient, some weeks before her admission to the Psychiatric Division).

Diagnosis

Giant urticaria and fainting found to be due to certain foods and to the propellant in aerosol sprays and other inhaled hydrocarbons e.g. motor car fumes.

Recommendation for future management

She should continue on her compatible diet and must avoid exposure to aerosol sprays and related chemicals such as car exhaust emissions, floor and furniture polishes, etc. She under-

stands this approach to her illness and will be followed up by
Dr Mackarness at his out-patient clinic.

Summary

A successful exercise in determining the causative allergens in a
resistant case of giant urticaria, complicated by fainting. Certain foods were incriminated, but the main offender turned out
to be the propellant in aerosol sprays and related hydrocarbons,
such as car exhaust fumes.

Prognosis

Hopeful if she avoids her specific allergens.

How common is this kind of case? Probably much more common
than most people think, judging by the way cases have been
appearing in popular newspapers and magazines. If someone said,
'False teeth would be impossible for me – my mouth would
ulcerate immediately' would you believe them? Mrs Shirley
Cleverdon, once a lecturer in English at a London College, talked
to Shelagh Massie of *Woman's Own*.[5] To most people, her illness
sounds so bizarre that they would have no hesitation in labelling
her neurotic or hysterical. Yet when you read her story, it carries
the ring of truth.

Not only plastic dentures upset her. She is made ill by the most
minute trace of almost any petrochemical or hydrocarbon with
which she comes in contact: car exhausts, cigarette smoke, floor
polishes, aerosol sprays . . . even her husband's after-shave. Her
symptoms began twenty years ago when she was thirty.

I remember one day when someone lit a cigarette thinking,
I don't like that. Then I began to find traffic fumes uncomfortable and I would go miles out of my way to avoid main roads.
After that I became conscious of deodorants and hair-sprays –
especially the aerosol kind.

The importance of the outside environment as a cause of ill-
health was first demonstrated in the case of infectious diseases
more than 100 years ago and the germ theory is now well ac-

cepted ... perhaps too well, judging by the freedom with which antibiotics are prescribed for the most trivial upsets, even for the common cold. By contrast, the other great group of illnesses caused by the physical environment – the allergies – although described since ancient times, are much less well understood by doctors and are largely neglected by research workers although, in developed countries today, I believe that allergy has surpassed infection as the number one cause of human ills.

Faced with patients with any kind of complaint, general practitioners and hospital doctors in the West first put them through a history-taking and diagnostic exclusion process so as not to miss underlying disordered anatomy or physiology together known as pathology. Signs of cancer or infection are looked for particularly.

When, finally, nothing is found to account for the patient's symptoms, often after long and costly investigations and referral to several specialists, heavy reassurance of the 'nothing physically wrong' variety is offered and the patient returned to the GP with prescriptions for drugs to suppress symptoms non-specifically. These prescriptions may then be repeated for a long time, resulting in home medicine cupboards becoming clogged with bottles of pills. In 1979 the *Daily Mail*[8] published a letter which shows how these repeat prescriptions can cumulate:

PILL AGE

Cleaning out an elderly lady's cupboards after she died, I found the following items of medication dating from between 1971 to the present day. Diconal: 20 bottles of 100; Distalgesic: 4 bottles of 100; Stemetil: 4 half bottles; Tuinal: 3 bottles of 200; Mogadon: 2 bottles part used; Lobak: 1 full bottle of 50; Orudis: 2 full bottles of 100; Intralgin Gel: 21 full tubes; Transvasin: 1 full tube; Anusol Suppositories: 4 full packets of 12; Hydrocortisone: one full tube; Spectacles in cases: 6. There were also various other part used bottles of tablets, some without labels. Is this why the Health Service costs so much?
(*Name and address supplied*)

I used this heavy drugging approach myself for seven years, from 1952 to 1959, in general practice at Kew in Surrey with a growing sense of failure and a feeling that I was somehow on the wrong track.

At this stage in my career, 1958, a trip to North America led to a meeting with Dr Ted Randolph in Chicago. He already had a unit at the Swedish Covenant Hospital, where he fasted patients on nothing but spring water in a chemical-free, non-polluted environment and demonstrated that under these conditions the same kinds of patient who were proving so difficult in my Kew practice could get well after 5 or 6 days and could have their symptoms brought back by challenges with single foods and chemicals which they had previously been swallowing or inhaling regularly.

The whole thing was a revelation to me and I could not wait to get back to England, try it out and write it up for other doctors to use. It certainly worked for some of my patients but persuading medical colleagues to take it seriously has taken another twenty years. In 1979 our top medical journal[27] ran a leading article which finally gave the approach respectability. Here is part of the last paragraph of that leader:

> Clearly, food intolerance can produce widespread symptoms in susceptible individuals, and many patients with troublesome and hitherto intractable symptoms can now be helped.[45] Some intriguing notions remain to be tested – notably the claim that certain foods may induce mental disease.[11] [23] [35] This idea dates back to at least Robert Burton's *Anatomy of Melancholy*.[2]

As a practising psychiatrist for fifteen years, I know that if food intolerance can affect the skin, the lungs or the blood vessels, producing diverse symptoms, there is no reason why, in some susceptible people, the brain should not be involved in an allergic reaction to a food additive, or a chemical in the air.

Dickens knew this, as was pointed out in *Harpers & Queen*,[22] by their health and beauty editor, Leslie Kenton, in a well-researched article on the chemistry of consciousness:

In Charles Dickens's *A Christmas Carol*, Jacob Marley, Scrooge's dead partner, appears to him as a ghost:

'You don't believe in me,' observed the Ghost. 'I don't,' said Scrooge. 'What evidence would you have of my reality beyond that of your senses?' 'I don't know,' said Scrooge. 'Why do you doubt your senses?' 'Because,' said Scrooge, 'a little thing affects them. A slight disorder of the stomach makes them cheats. You may be an undigested bit of beef, a blot of mustard, a crumb of cheese, a fragment of an underdone potato. There's more of gravy than of grave about you, whatever you are!'

Scrooge in his wisdom (even back in 1843) well knew that chemical changes in the body brought about by something one has eaten can affect the central nervous system and alter the consciousness enough to produce hallucinations or imaginary fears. Today, however, thanks to several generations of psychologically oriented doctors influenced by Freud's theory that mental illness occurs only as a result of early conditioning or trauma (the something-nasty-in-the-woodshed theory), medical science is only just rediscovering this truth. But it is a discovery that is likely to transform the whole face of psychology and psychiatry in the next twenty years. Strong evidence is emerging that such diverse mental and emotional conditions as schizophrenia, manic depression, anxiety and uncontrolled aggression are primarily chemical in origin – the results of allergic reactions to food or pollutants, deficiencies in the body of one or more trace minerals, toxic poisoning from heavy metals such as lead, or combinations of all three.

I first published a paper on food and chemical allergy in 1959[32] and here are the conclusions I drew from my first four cases treated by elimination dieting:

The difficulty of treating patients disabled with psychosomatic or functional* disorders on psychiatric lines in general practice

*'Functional' means with no demonstrable pathology. It is often used in a dismissive way by doctors with the implication that the patient is not really ill.

has led me to experiment with possible non-psychiatric ways of tackling these problem patients. So far, a dietetic approach has been the most successful. Using it, I have been able to rehabilitate four patients: two men, a woman and a boy all of whom were so seriously disabled by their symptoms that they could neither work effectively nor enjoy life.

Their complaints differed widely. The woman had chronic abdominal pain, the boy a behaviour disorder so severe that he was unmanageable at home and unteachable at school. Of the two men, one had pain of the peptic ulcer syndrome type, vomiting and Ménière-like giddiness; the other a disabling travel-phobia, obesity depression, periodic bouts of diarrhoea and other psychosomatic symptoms. In three of the four cases, hospitals had failed to do more than tie the functional label on more tightly.

This was my clinical material. Unpromising perhaps when viewed from the popular psychiatric 'it's-all-due-to-emotional-conflict' angle, but nevertheless four people who were ill in the real sense of the word. So ill that their lives was miserable and dominated by their symptoms.

An interest in obesity led me to write a little monograph[33] two years ago in which I criticized the current idea that over-weight was due primarily to over-nutrition. I came to the con-clusion that more fat people became fat for metabolic reasons than because they ate too much, and the diet which I described proved to be one which enabled fat people to become thinner while still eating as much as they liked. In general terms, this diet was high-fat, high-protein, low-carbohydrate and un-restricted calorie.

Food Allergy and Disease

While in Canada and the United States at the end of 1958, I met a number of doctors who had read my book and who told me that they thought the diet worked for reasons different from the ones I gave. 'It works,' they said, 'because you warn fat people off the food to which they are commonly allergic. Obesity is a manifestation of allergy.'

This was a new idea to me and I listened with great interest. The story goes back to work done in the late 1920s and early 1930s by an American allergist, Dr Albert Rowe[49]. He drew attention to the importance of food and chemical allergy as a factor in many common diseases and advocated the use of elimination diets as a means of identifying and excluding the foods responsible. In his opinion, most food allergies are to substances in the carbohydrate group, particularly wheat and corn products. He showed that skin tests are misleading as a means of identifying such allergens.

These views led him into conflict with orthodox allergists who believed that if an allergen could not be identified by skin tests based on the antigen/antibody reaction (see p 33), then the condition it was suspected of causing was not allergic. Despite this, several allergists, including Arthur Coca, Herbert J. Rinkel and Théron G. Randolph, have used modifications of his methods with success. I stayed with Randolph for a few days in Chicago last December and spent time on his wards at the Swedish Covenant Hospital. What I saw there convinced me that food allergy might be the key to a number of resistant cases among my own patients.

Having no hospital at my disposal, I could not use Randolph's method of taking patients into a ward especially screened for allergens, starving them for five days, feeding them foods singly at intervals through the day and observing their reactions clinically, biochemically and pathologically with the help of technicians, a good nursing staff and a dietician. I had to adapt the method to an NHS practice without ancillary help. This led me to evolve what I now call the Stone Age Regime.

The Stone Age diet, which I still use in my hospital clinic for patients who for one reason or another find it impossible to go on a total fast, is based on fresh meat, fish, fowl, vegetables and fruit, with only non-chlorinated spring water to drink. It is continued for four or five days, until symptoms clear. If symptoms do not clear or do not improve considerably, then the diagnosis

of food allergy must be questioned, or inhaled chemicals suspected. Symptoms from these will not go unless the patient is
kept in a chemically clean environment, which is not easy to
provide in a modern gas-heated and plastic-furnished home or
hospital.

The rest of my paper on the Stone Age diet gave some of my
thoughts and conclusions about the ecological approach to
mysterious modern illnesses. Twenty years' subsequent experience in clinical ecology has not made me change these opinions.

Discussion

Perhaps it is too soon to try to draw any conclusions from these
cases. It could be argued that the apparent improvement in
each is no more than could be expected to result from any form
of enthusiastic attention. However, the case of the boy of seven,
whom I dealt with via his mother and took care not to see until
after he got better, is against this explanation. And perhaps it is
significant that, on the one hand, the foods which caused no
symptoms in all four cases were those unprocessed foods to
which we have been adapted for longest in our evolutionary
history: meats of all kinds, dairy fats, eggs, milk and fruit;
while on the other, the foods which caused the worst reactions
were the refined cereals and the canned, preserved and frozen
packaged foods to which we have only recently been heavily
exposed.

Self-help

Some may consider an elimination diet tedious to conduct, but
in fact few types of treatment are so interesting or so kind to
the doctor/patient relationship. It is a joint effort requiring real
co-operation from the patient, who can feel involved in solving
his own problem.

I think my Stone Age modification of Randolph's regime is
a legitimate short cut which starts the patient off by eliminating
all those things which have recently come into our food and
which, if the theory is right, are causing the trouble by confronting our cells with substances with which they are ill-equipped
to deal biochemically, not being adapted to them. Of course

there are no foods which have never caused a reaction in any-body, and for this reason the patient must be exposed to foods singly at first, though later new foods may be added, one at a time, to other foods already proved to be safe. All I am doing with the Stone Age diet is to cut out a whole group of common allergens before starting. The method is not unscientific and can be made to conform to a set of postulates like Koch's*:

1 Withholding all food must be shown to result in clinical improvement.

2 Eating foods found to be 'safe on testing' must not cause symptoms.

3 Test-feeding known allergenic foods, singly or together, must bring back the symptoms.

Conclusions

Many theories have been put forward to account for the increase in the number of patients with neurosis and psychosomatic illness today. Psychiatrists have persistently claimed that they have the secret, but somehow they have failed to give the GP a solution he can use. I do not think we are being subjected to much more psychological stress now than we were twenty-five years ago, but I am sure that the sophistication and adulteration of food with chemical additives has increased enormously in that time and so has the consumption of processed starch and sugar (white bread, cakes, biscuits, sweets and soft drinks).

*In 1876 Robert Koch, a German bacteriologist and discoverer of the tuberculosis bacterium, had set out three criteria or postulates which must be fulfilled if evidence of a causal connection between an illness and a bacterial infection is to be accepted as valid:

1 The bacterium is to be demonstrated in all cases.

2 Its distribution in the body must correspond with the parts affected: e.g. ulcer, glands or spots.

3 The micro-organism must be recoverable and capable of being grown on a suitable culture medium outside the body.

For food and chemical allergy to become acceptable scientifically, criteria such as these must be met.

It would be surprising if people were not allergic to pesticides put into the ground and sprayed on crops, to flour 'improvers', anti-staling agents, emulsifying compounds, artificial colourings, preservatives and the whole terrifying array of potentially toxic substances now being added to our food in order to improve its appearance, flavour, shelf-life and profitability.

Summary
Food allergy as a cause of disease, particularly the role of processed cereal foods as allergens, is described. An account is given of the treatment of four cases of disabling psychosomatic disorder on non-psychiatric lines, using a Stone Age (pre-cereal) elimination diet.

The implications of the increasing use of chemical food additives are briefly discussed.

It is clear that the early clinical ecologists were more concerned with allergy to foods than to chemicals, and it was not until the late 1950s and early 1960s that Chicago allergist Dr Ted Randolph began publishing methods of demonstrating the cause-and-effect relationship between exposure to environmental chemicals and many common relapsing illnesses of unknown cause. But in spite of a growing following among doctors acquainted with his work, chemical agents in food, drink and ambient air (particularly indoor air pollution) are still rarely considered as probable precipitators of the common symptoms which plague civilized man.

Vets and farmers always look to the diet and other aspects of the physical surroundings when an animal is off colour, but few modern doctors consider the possibility that the patient may be showing signs of adaptive breakdown in the face of a food or other physical substances in the environment.

If any abnormality is found, efforts are made to restore things to normal with drugs or surgical operations or, if that is not possible, the malfunctioning organ is sometimes cut away. Above all, drugs are given for everything, whether underlying pathology has been established or not. The most important thing on which doctors and patients now seem to agree is to try to find a magic drug, which will strike home to the seat of the trouble within the body and set things right.

All this is a long way from the Hippocratic tradition to which doctors are still supposed to pay lip service in their Hippocratic oath, which, among other things, requires that the doctor do his patient no harm. Central to the Hippocratic tradition was the idea that natural forces re-establish health in the sick body if the right food and environment is provided.

Here is another case which I saw demonstrated when I visited Dr William Rea's Environmental Control Unit in Dallas for the first time in November 1977. It is typical of the hundreds he has treated on similar lines since his twenty-bed unit (now expanded to forty beds) was set up in 1975.

In her job at a semiconductor plastic factory, Mrs A, a 53-year-old white female, mixed a variety of dry chemicals (sodium hyposulphate, ammonium sulphate, ammonium chloride and nickel) into solution. She had worked at this job for approximately three years without symptoms. During this period she was breathing the fumes of these chemicals as well as those of the plastics. Her symptoms began with one month of malaise after an accidental over-exposure to the chemical powders and synthetic solutions. The malaise gradually worsened when she was at work but improved when she was away from the factory. Later, symptoms consisting of irritation in the nose, otitis, ringing in the ears and hoarseness developed in the upper respiratory tract. Symptoms progressed to disabling nasal and ear problems and aphonia which was treated by an otolaryngologist*. The doctor recommended that she stay away from work for a period of time. As soon as she felt improved, she returned to work but was unable to obtain better ventilation around the chemicals and again became ill with sinusitis. Again, she stayed away from work and felt better. Then she was moved to another part of the factory but still inhaled ambient chemicals in the air. This time she developed wheezing,

*A specialist in ear, nose and throat.

spontaneous bruising, gastro-intestinal upset, skin rashes, and an inability to concentrate.

At this point, Mrs A entered the Environmental Unit for chemical incitant testing.

Her symptoms cleared in four days, at which time food challenges with chemically less contaminated food produced no symptoms. With inhalation chemical challenges, a transient exposure to polyester clothing gave immediate hoarseness, followed by watering eyes which lasted thirty minutes. Wearing permanent pressed clothing for one hour caused a stuffy nose, closed eustachian tubes, and a dry cough which lasted for six hours. A ten-minute exposure to nylon caused facial flushing and itching which lasted twenty minutes. The odour of ordinary tap water when exposed while drawing for a bath caused headache, while ingestion of one glass produced a stomach ache and extreme bloating. Chlorine odour challenge derived from fumes coming from diluted Chlorox didthe same. Additives in commercial foods triggered confusion, bloating, nausea, headache, spontaneous bruising, and depression. Inhalation of Raid insecticide at ordinary ambient concentrations* produced nausea, confusion, loss of equilibrium, and a dry cough. Fumes from the flames of a well-functioning gas stove caused lightheadedness, swollen glands, earache, sore throat and pressure in the head. After discharge, the patient was placed on a rotary diversified diet† of less chemically contaminated foods and instructed to drink only spring water, and to avoid chemicals which would incite her problem. Although the patient is now avoiding petrochemically contaminated situations and is steadily improving, one year after withdrawal from this contaminated environment she still cannot work in her previous job.

*Ambient concentrations. The amount of a chemical substance in the air accepted as safe by commercial and governmental agencies.
†A diet which rotates permitted foods through a three to five day cycle, so that no food is taken too often. Frequent resort to the same foods, meal after meal and day after day, has been found to create new allergies, making an already limited diet still more restrictive (see appendix D).

An important general point for students of chemical allergy comes out of this quotation from Professor Rea. In this case and in others he showed me, it seems that a massive dose of one chemical sensitized the patients not only to that particular one, but rendered them more susceptible to others. He calls this the spreading phenomenon and I have observed it in cases I have had under my care. Once this spreading occurs, reactions follow upon minute exposures to other chemical contaminants of food, air and water.

It is not too fanciful to suppose that the first, single massive dose breaches the patient's immune defences so that thereafter even tiny doses can enter their bodies and cause unpleasant reactions. At any rate, that is what seemed to happen to a patient of mine, Miss C. H. who suffered her first massive exposure to chemicals in the great smog which blanketed London in the winter of 1952, killing thousands of people susceptible to respiratory illness (bronchitis and the like).

Before the passing of the Clean Air Act, as a direct consequence of this lethal 1952 smog, chimneys in British towns and cities were allowed to pour smoke containing corrosive gases into the atmosphere. Fog would descend from time to time, bringing droplets of water in which these corrosive gases would dissolve to form sulphuric and other acids, strong enough to eat away the stone of which ancient monuments like Westminster Abbey are built. What these acids did to the lungs of people who inhaled them is not difficult to imagine.

Miss C. H. was stranded at Marble Arch and had to get to Shepherd's Bush, about four miles away. There was no transport, so she walked. By the time she got home she had asthma from which she has suffered ever since and for which she has been given steroids. It is triggered by the smallest chemical exposure.

I can remember that 1952 smog. I had just started my general practice at Kew Gardens, seven miles from the centre of London. To do a house call to an acutely ill patient I had to tie a wet cloth over my nose and mouth and find the way by feeling with my hand along the walls bordering the roads, relying on my sense of direction to get me there and back. The smog was a dirty yellow-green colour, tasted vile and was so thick that I could not see my own feet.

At this stage, before I have side-tracked the reader with too much anecdotal material, I want to make clear what the central theme and purpose of this book is.

It is to try to find an answer to the most puzzling, paradoxical, far reaching problem facing modern man: why, in spite of unprecedented technical progress and know-how and the expenditure of vast and ever-increasing sums of money on health services, does good health continue to elude us in middle age? And why are modern doctors still unable to explain much of what ails us or apply effective remedies?

To be logical and scientific about it, this problem which affects us all, whether we happen to be sick or well at the moment, should be tackled under five headings:

1 Hypothesis or theory as to the cause of the problem.
2 Experiments designed to test the chosen hypothesis.
3 Predicted results of these experiments.
4 Observed results of the experiments.
5 Conclusions to be drawn from these results.

The hypothesis I am going to examine in this book is that man has inherited a stone-age body and psychology, with powers of adaptation superior to those of any other animal but unequal to the task of adapting to the rapid changes in his diet and physical environment that have occurred since the industrial revolution. Such a hypothesis is testable by the techniques of clinical ecology and I shall give the results of some of the more important of these experiments which have been carried out so far, not only by me but by doctors in other parts of the world.

Support for this hypothesis is not hard to find for it appeals to many observant people as reasonable and worth investigating further.

Our food is the part of our environment with which we come into closest contact. After digestion and absorption it enters the blood stream and is carried to every cell in the body, not just as fuel to supply warmth and the energy for movement, but to supply the building blocks for growth when we are young, to repair worn out and damaged tissues and to furnish the genetic material with which we hand on life to our offspring. Fresh, good quality food is as essential to health as clean air and pure water. We tamper with it at our peril.

Yet, with scarcely a murmur of protest, we have allowed the food of the American and British people to be transformed and polluted to an extent unimaginable to our grandparents. Professor Ross Hume Hall, who runs a course on the nature of industrialized society at McMaster University, Hamilton, Ontario, Canada, in his book *Food for Nought* [16]:

... a highly individual system of growing and marketing food has been transformed into a gigantic, highly integrated service system, in which the object is not to nourish or even to feed, but to force an ever-increasing consumption of fabricated products. This phenomenon is not peculiar to the American scene and occurs in every industrialized country. The United States, however, has progressed furthest in the transformation. Man can never be more than what he eats, and one would expect that a phenomenon with such profound effects on health and well-being as a radical system of supplying nourishment would be thoroughly documented and assessed by the scientific community. Such is not the case. The transformation has gone unmarked by government agencies and learned bodies. Government agencies, recipients of the public trust, charged with protecting and improving the public's food, operate as if the technology of food fabrication rested in pre-World War II days. Scientific bodies, supported by public funds and charged with assessing and improving the public's health, ignore completely the results of contemporary methods of producing and marketing foods.

What are those results? There is growing evidence from epidemiology, anthropology, biochemistry, pathology and clinical medicine to show that the results are leading to disaster.

The disaster which I and my colleagues in clinical ecology predict for industrialized man could still be forestalled by resolute, far-sighted action by individuals and ultimately by government departments responsible for regulating the food supply and the environment.

There is no need for us to pollute ourselves out of existence. Seventy million years ago, the dinosaurs found their environment changed as suddenly as ours is changing this century. Lacking our intelligence and technical accomplishments, their fate was a foregone conclusion. Ours is not ... yet, anyway.

Long ago, when man's remote mammalian ancestors were tiny, shrew-like creatures living in burrows, hot-blooded dinosaurs ruled the earth for 170 million years. They lived either in swamps, browsing all day on the copious vegetation, or as swift-footed, predatory carnivores, running on two powerful hind legs, as ostriches do now, and eating the flesh of the herbivores. Suddenly, they disappeared within not much more than 100 years. We do not yet know what hit them. Theories abound; among the more likely, a cataclysmic, nearby stellar explosion which changed the climate of the earth in seconds.

Whatever the cause of the change in climate, the plant food withered. No longer able to get the minerals from the plants with which to build their huge bones the dinosaurs became extinct, leaving the birds to become their only direct descendants today. The sufferings of the dinosaurs are unimaginable, but is there a lesson in their fate for late twentieth century man?

Half the known extinctions of species since the first recorded one in about 80 AD (the European lion) have occurred in our own century. Eric Eckholm, writing for the Worldwatch Institute, says that the next few years will see an even greater holocaust – not only of birds and animals but of plants, molluscs and insects of vital importance to the well-being of man.

A good example is what happened in Borneo when they introduced insecticides to kill the mosquitos which carry the malarial parasite; the insecticides accumulated in cockroaches, most of which are resistant to insecticides. Geckoes (lizards with sticky feet which enable them to run upside down) fed on the cockroaches, became lethargic and fell prey to cats.

The cats died, rats multiplied and with the rats came the threat to the native population of leptospirosis and bubonic plague (once epidemic in England as the Black Death) and the army had to parachute more cats into the jungle villages.

As long ago as 1943, when he retired as Conservator of Forests for the Indian province of Assam, my father told me that pressure from local politicians was eroding the conservation of the forests of North-East India to which he had devoted his life. For a monetary consideration, Assamese box-wallahs were being allowed to take wood out of the jungle, with no thought for the future of the elephants, tigers and rhino which are now becoming extinct.

Wildlife ecologist Norman Myers says that one species is disappearing every day in tropical forests alone and that in a few more years there may be a species lost every hour.

Nearly all the food we eat comes from only about twenty crops while thousands of plants are edible and some would form valuable additions to our diet, particularly useful to those patients who have become allergic to most of the limited ingredients in modern foods and are looking for new alternatives. Types of trees which could be developed as sources of industrial products, from medicines to building materials, are being wiped out.

Our early mammalian ancestors were not subjected to this concentrated destruction and pollution of their habitat. They could eat almost anything; animal or vegetable. They were small enough to hide from early predatory birds and other enemies and eventually, after millions more years, they evolved into apes, apemen and finally modern man. By discovering fire, man survived the ice ages, and by inventing more and more ingenious weapons and co-operative ways of hunting, he came to dominate the earth as the dinosaurs had done before him.

But what now? Our physical environment, including our food, is changing almost as quickly as it did all those millions of years ago. In the last 6,000 years, we have gone over from meat to a diet based on cereal grains. 'What is wrong with that?' ask the vegetarians. Very little, so long as we eat the cereals in their original form, unprocessed and unrefined; but do we?

We shall look at the way our food, including cereal grains, has been adulterated during recent years by the addition of chemicals, preservatives and additives later on in this book.

TWO

The discovery of allergy

Most illnesses, apart from infections, were thought by the nineteenth century doctors who pioneered scientific medicine to have arisen from faults within the body or the mind, and are still thought to do so. The bulk of teaching in our medical schools follows this premise with the result that modern treatment is aimed at correcting supposed anatomical or biochemical defects by means of surgical operations and drugs.

Girls who are embarrassed by heavy sweating (one of the commonest symptoms of allergy to certain foods and chemicals) are sent to surgeons who painstakingly remove the sweat glands from their armpits. Men complaining of day-long fatigue and low spirits for no good reason, after a batch of X-rays and blood tests have all come back normal, usually end up with the psychiatrist who, although he may think the complaint is all in the patient's mind, will prescribe mood-altering drugs designed to correct abnormalities of brain chemistry.

Heart transplants – spectacular and often successful in the short term – are a ludicrously expensive and labour-intensive way of dealing with heart disease brought about by environmental factors[45] which have damaged not only the heart but all the blood vessels in the victim's body. For the cost of one heart transplant, hundreds of hyperactive children could be calmed down and brought back to normal with appropriate ecological treatment and advice, rather than doomed to failure at school.

The importance of the outside physical environment as a cause of ill-health was first demonstrated in infectious diseases more than 100 years ago and the germ theory is now well accepted. The other great group of illnesses caused by the physical environment – the allergies – although recognized and described since ancient times, are much less well understood by doctors and largely neglected by research workers, although it has been estimated that in developed countries today, allergy has surpassed infection as the number one cause of human ills.

Since 1873 when the first experimental observations on the link between pollen and hay fever were published, allergy has gradually divided into two streams, one following the work of Clemens von Pirquet[39], the Viennese paediatrician who first coined the word 'allergy' in 1906 and defined it as 'an acquired, specific, altered capacity to react to physical substances on the part of the tissues of the body', and the other following the science of immunology which was concerned with the internal bio-chemical mechanisms on which immunity (resistance) to germs, toxins and other environmental factors depend.

Von Pirquet's wide, biological view of allergy, formulated before precise details of immunological mechanisms had been worked out, led eventually to a school of allergists who call themselves clinical ecologists and take an exogenous (generated from outside) view of allergy, concentrating on identifying and eliminating environmental factors. They regard this aspect of allergy as most important and in the long run more helpful to the patient who is spared the ingestion of powerful, synthetic drugs and their unavoidable and often nasty side-effects.

Immunological allergists, who now dominate teaching and research in allergy, have focused more and more on endogenous (internally generated) processes, which has led to the development of injectable protective vaccines and to the use of drugs such as antihistamines and steroids (cortisone-like compounds) to suppress allergic symptoms non-specifically. Little effort is made by them to identify, measure, eliminate or avoid the substances in the environment which give rise to the allergic symptoms.

By generally accepted definition, allergy means an unusual or altered response to contact with a substance foreign to the body. Today, in developed countries, nearly everyone has some sort of allergy or knows someone who has.

For a long time, these two schools of allergists were working apart, each claiming that theirs was the better approach. Today they are starting to work together and a third group of allergists is growing in importance; the clinical immunologists, who admit that there are aspects of allergy not yet explainable in terms of biochemistry, which are recognizable clinically and in which the underlying biological processes need to be worked out, so that rational treatment may be applied. Clinical immunology flourishes as a research subject and cannot be divorced from laboratory research, but cross-fertilization between laboratory and clinic is the lifeblood of immunology and it is in gaining immunological know-how that clinical ecology will evolve and become more widely accepted in medicine.

There have always been certain people who show intolerance for specific constituents of their physical environment. Hippocrates mentioned them in his writings 400 years before Christ, and in Roman times Lucretius wrote, '*Quod aliis cibus est aliis fuat acra venarum*' (what's food for some may be fierce poison for others). This quotation is usually translated as 'one man's meat is another man's poison'.

So, long before the word allergy was invented, it was recognized that some unlucky people were made ill by eating, drinking, touching, inhaling things which the majority could take without untoward reaction.

The scientific study of idiosyncracy began in 1873, when Dr Charles Blackley [4], a London physician, first published observations made on himself and a group of fellow hay fever sufferers which showed that minute quantities of pollen placed in the nose could provoke an attack.

Food allergy did not attract serious medical attention until about fifty years later when, in the 1920s, Dr Albert Rowe, an allergist in California, began using diets which excluded one group of foods at a time in order to identify those which were causing his patients' migraines, recurring asthma, colitis and other chronic disorders. Rowe was treated with hostility by most of his medical colleagues but attracted a small number of interested and open-minded doctors who went on to expand the work which he had started and to found the Society for Clinical Ecology in 1965.

After meeting Rowe, Dr Herbert Rinkel of Kansas City

developed the individual provocative food ingestion test in the late 1930s which he presented at a medical meeting in 1941. Instead of cutting out families of foods (see appendix E) from his patients' diets, as Rowe had done, Rinkel made them leave out one food at a time – choosing the ones they seemed to like best – then if they lost their symptoms after five or six days he would ask them back to his office to eat a portion of the avoided food as a test and to see if their symptoms returned acutely.

He had developed this technique in working out his own allergy to eggs, which had caused him much trouble with headaches and nasal symptoms as a student and young doctor. From these original observations, Rinkel discovered the phenomenon of masking, a key concept in the understanding of food and chemical allergy. He defined it thus: 'If one uses a food every day or so, one may be allergic to it but never suspect it as a cause of symptoms. It is common to feel better after a meal at which the food is used than before mealtime. This is called masked food allergy.'

Masking explained why many American clinical ecologists now refer to food allergy as food addiction. The continual eating of a food to which allergy has developed will, sometimes for many years, keep the patient feeling good; *so long as that food is taken often*, preferably at every meal. Omission of the food for a day or two will bring on withdrawal or hangover symptoms, curable by resort to more of the same food. The analogy with alcoholism and drug addiction is obvious and in fact most alcoholics and drug addicts are chemical victims of allergy to the poison on which they have become hooked.

Recently a case was reported to me on one of the wards at the hospital which illustrates well this masking and pick-up effect.

Sharon was in the ward under the care of another psychiatrist who was giving her tranquillizers and anti-depressants to combat suicidal thoughts and frequent bouts of unbearable nervous tension. A patient of mine who shared a four-bed dormitory with this unhappy girl remarked to me how often Sharon sprayed her hair with lacquer – every hour or more often if she was feeling particularly tense. The spraying seemed to calm her down for a short time.

Most modern aerosol hair sprays consist of a lacquer, such as shellac, and perfume dissolved in a petrochemical solvent which also acts as the propellant when the nozzle is pressed. The propellant is a fluorocarbon, related to carbon tetrachloride, the solvent in dry cleaning fluid. Fluorocarbons are chemicals in an unstable phase between liquid and gas. Under pressure in the can they are liquid but on release into the air through the nozzle they escape as gas which carries with it very fine droplets of the fluorocarbon in which the lacquer and perfume are dissolved. These tiny droplets can be inhaled deep into the lungs so that their constituent chemicals enter the blood stream and reach the brain where they may set up allergic and/or toxic reactions which manifest as depression or abnormal behaviour in susceptible people. Like glue-sniffing (see p 124), hair spray inhalation can become addictive.

Freudian psychiatrists would probably find some convoluted explanation for Sharon's addiction to the hair spray, but having treated many cases of allergy to petrochemicals I suspect that this girl was a chemical allergy victim and was using her chance discovery of masking to relieve some of her symptoms, although she never came under my care.

One of the earliest papers about chemical fumes causing allergy appeared in 1954 in the *Annals of Allergy*, under the title, 'The asthmathogenic effects of odors, smells and fumes'.[3] This allergic effect of chemical inhalants was regarded as a rarity until 1962 when Dr Ted Randolph published his now well-known book [44] which has become a source book for clinical ecologists and is now accepted as a landmark on the road to better understanding of allergic disease, even by some orthodox allergists.

As recently as November 1978, at the Twelfth Advanced Seminar in Clinical Ecology, held by the Society for Clinical Ecology in Florida, one of the guest speakers was Professor Jack Pepys, Director of the Department of Clinical Immunology at the Cardiothoracic Institute, Brompton Hospital, London. His subject 'Respiratory Allergic Diseases due to Environmental Chemical Agents'. Professor Pepys is the doyen of British clinical immunologists and a world authority on the biochemical mechanisms underlying allergy. He told the meeting how and why chemical fumes in tiny amounts can cause asthma in susceptible people and I would guess that within a year or two, the medical profession as a whole will stop dismissing chemical victims as hysterical or psychosomatic and start accepting them for what they are – casualties in the battle to adapt to pollutants in both food and environment. Sufferers deserve all the skilled help our hospitals and GPs can give.

To understand the terms ecology and immunology more fully, it is helpful to go back in time and look at how man has adapted to his environment and survived.

Man is at the head of the animal kingdom because he is the most adaptable of all living creatures and so has thrived under widely differing physical conditions for millions of years. Prehistoric remains and ancient history strongly suggest that disease has always been a part of human life, but from bones and skulls it is evident that few early men were old when they died, so their pattern of disease is not strictly comparable with our own.

The anthropological evidence indicates that life under the most uncomfortable conditions is compatible with good health. But the ability to adapt to any sort of environment, however hostile, depends on that environment remaining stable. At the time of their discovery by white men, primitive people like the Polynesians, Eskimos and American Indians had all lived in stable, almost unchanging physical and social environments for centuries.

They had achieved equilibrium with their food supplies, climate and natural surroundings and had developed a high level of immunity to those germs prevalent among them. This immunity soon broke down when their isolated communities were infiltrated by explorers and traders.

The pattern has always been the same. Soon after meeting the Europeans, these primitive people went down with devastating epidemics of infectious diseases such as measles, whooping cough and tuberculosis caused by microbes which the Europeans carried and to which most of them were immune. The process worked in reverse too. British settlers moving into India in Victorian times were killed in large numbers by malaria and dysentery which the native population resisted with greater success because of acquired immunity to local strains of the causative micro-organisms.

Against this historical background of the interaction of explorers with isolated, stable communities of primitive people, it is easy to see how interest in ecology and immunity arose. The scientists and doctors wanted information from explorers and at the time when Charles Darwin (1809–82) formulated his theory of evolution a contemporary German biologist, Ernst Haeckel,[15] first used the word ecology in 1866 to mean the inter-relationships between living organisms and their environments. (He took the word from the Greek *oikos* = living place and *logos* = knowledge.)

The invention of the microscope enabled the French chemist Louis Pasteur (1822–95) to demonstrate the role of very small living cells (bacteria) in the causation of disease. Pasteur went on to prove that animals could be immunized or protected against disease-causing bacteria. He first protected sheep against anthrax.

Anthrax is an acute, infectious disease of animals which causes blood poisoning and congestion of the lungs. It is transmissable to man either as a lung infection known as wool-sorters disease or as a slow-growing, spreading skin pustule which, unless treated, can lead to septicaemia and death. Pasteur had identified abnormal, rod-shaped cells in the blood from sheep recently dead from anthrax, under his microscope. He showed that the cells were alive by growing them at blood heat (37°C) on agar, a nutrient medium, on which in twelve hours they formed visible colonies like locks of wavy hair. Next, he injected quantities of these abnormal rod-shaped cells (or bacilli) into healthy sheep and found that they soon died of anthrax. The idea of protecting sheep against anthrax by injecting them with attenuated or weakened anthrax bacilli came to Pasteur from earlier work done by a Gloucestershire GP, Edward Jenner (1749–1823).

In Jenner's time, it was estimated that every tenth person in Europe died of smallpox. In 1760, the disease killed 24,234 people in London, out of a total population of 650,000. Most of those who survived were ugly with pock-marks, some scarred for life. As he did his rounds in Gloucestershire from farm to farm, Jenner was able to confirm with his own eyes the truth of the local folklore that dairy maids who caught cowpox, a much milder disease, from the udders of infected cows were immune to smallpox.

Jenner, like other British and Continental doctors, was using a method called variolation against smallpox. It involved trying to give the patient a non-fatal attack of smallpox in order to confer immunity, by inoculating the skin with matter from a pustule on an actual case of the disease. It was already known that one attack of a contagious disease protected against another, and recovered cases of smallpox were used to nurse new victims.

The method had originated in the Far East and in 1718 Lady Mary Wortly Montagu brought the idea back to England from Constantinople, where her husband had been British ambassador. She had had her own children protected by a Greek physician and they had survived. Variolation caused some deaths, however, and the main objection to it was that inoculated people were infectious and could and did spread smallpox.

Putting these things together, Jenner wondered whether cowpox might be a mild, animal form of smallpox and whether inoculation with the lesser disease might protect against the more lethal smallpox or *variola major* as doctors called it. He put the idea to the test on 14 May 1796 when he inoculated an eight-year-old boy, James Phipps, with pus taken from a cowpox blister on the hand of a milkmaid. The boy developed a mild attack of cowpox and recovered. On 1 July, Jenner inoculated the child again, this time with real smallpox. Nothing happened. Three months later he repeated it, but the boy resisted the disease. Convinced now beyond reasonable doubt that the method was safe and effective, Jenner decided to publish his findings and wrote a paper for the Royal Society. The learned members were not impressed. They returned his paper – standard behaviour for entrenched pundits in any walk of life when faced with anything new.

This did not put Jenner off. In 1798 he published a book about his work,[20] '*An enquiry into the causes and effects of variolae vaccinae*' (*vacca* is the Latin for cow and it is from this use of the word vaccination by Jenner that all protective inoculations have come to be called vaccines).

He put forward the theory that man and certain animals had become alike through living together and that therefore it was not unreasonable to imagine an animal disease such as cowpox giving protection against a similar human disease like smallpox. He gave a well-reasoned account of his theory. It sounded good, but in fact he had got it all wrong.

He thought cowpox began in horses, was transferred to the udders of cows by grooms and then from the cows' udders to the hands of milkmaids and cowmen. It didn't matter, because vaccination with cowpox worked. It really did protect people from smallpox and it was a safe procedure, unlike Lady Mary Wortly Montagu's variolation, once widely practised throughout Europe and Asia and declared illegal in England in 1840.

Jenner's method of vaccination was adopted all over the civilized world, but after some years opposition to it grew as more and more cases of smallpox in vaccinated persons were reported. The need for periodic re-vaccination to maintain immunity was soon appreciated, but right up to his death in 1823, Jenner never recognized the necessity for it and stubbornly tried to make excuses for every case of failure he came across.

With no laboratories at his disposal, Jenner had no inkling as to how vaccination worked. As a GP he was an observant and courageous clinician. The grateful British government awarded him £30,000 (a huge sum in those days). Napoleon insisted that his troops be vaccinated.

Mesmerized by our advanced technology today, we are in danger of forgetting the debt we owe to Jenner. Present neglect of vaccination and indifference to the closure of smallpox research laboratories following the Birmingham tragedy in 1978 may bring smallpox raging back to Europe and America within the next decade.

To return to Pasteur, he had shown that he could give sheep anthrax with an injection of some of the little rod-shaped bacilli grown from the blood of an infected sheep. From Jenner's work, Pasteur reasoned that if cowpox vaccination could protect against virulent smallpox, then if he could injure but not kill his anthrax bacilli they might no longer kill sheep but protect them. He had already noted that old cultures of chicken cholera germs would not cause the expected disease when injected into healthy chickens. This reduction of virulence was called attenuation.

So Pasteur took fifty healthy sheep and vaccinated half of them with attenuated anthrax bacilli. Two weeks later, on 31 May 1881, all fifty were given injections of virulent anthrax bacilli. Two days later, twenty-two of the unvaccinated sheep lay dead. Two more were dying and the twenty-fifth died that night. The twenty-five vaccinated sheep remained well. The infant science of immunology was on its way.

Pasteur's experiment showed conclusively that Jenner's success in vaccination against smallpox must have been due to the inoculation of the same germ, or a closely related one, with its virulence diminished. *In the interval between the first injection of the harmless vaccine and the final injection of the virulent germ, which later investigation showed must be ten days or more, the cells of the body must have developed some way of protecting themselves against the harmful environmental influence of deadly germs. They had immunized themselves.*

It is not surprising that Jenner, working one hundred years before Pasteur, with nothing but his GP's common sense to guide him, should not have had much idea how vaccination worked.

This story illustrates the link between clinical observations (Jenner) and laboratory-based experimentation (Pasteur). They need each other in order to allow medical advances to gain acceptance and be put to practical use. Without Jenner's brilliant deductions about smallpox and cowpox and his daring in putting his ideas to the test, Pasteur might never have thought of attenuating anthrax bacilli and using them to protect sheep. Nor might he have gone on to repeat his success with rabies, against which terrible disease a modification of his vaccine is still used today to save people from death after being bitten by a rabid dog.

Other investigators soon developed vaccines against typhoid, cholera, diphtheria and tuberculosis. By 1900, following the discovery of antitoxins to neutralize the deadly toxins or poisons produced by disease-causing germs when they multiply in the body, it became possible not only to prevent people from catching most of the infectious diseases, but to treat them effectively even if they became infected. Antitoxins led to a more effective treatment, chemotherapy (drugs to knock out germs without harming the patient), and finally to antibiotics (penicillin and the rest of the mould-derived germ killers) which completed the conquest of infectious disease which had been the greatest threat to life before these remedies were found.

Doctors wanted to know how Pasteur's immunization worked. How did the cells of which the human body is composed protect themselves against germs? The answer was provided by Paul Ehrlich (1854–1915), German chemist and physician, discoverer of Salvarsan, the first effective chemotherapeutic drug against syphilis. Interested in the prevention and cure of infection by chemical means, Ehrlich began by studying the action of aniline dyes and their effects on diseases in animals. His first success was the discovery of a dye which was active against the protozoal micro-organism, *Trypanosoma gambiense*, which is carried by the tsetse fly and causes sleeping sickness. It was natural for Ehrlich to suggest a theory of immunity expressed in chemical terms. He knew that the chemical basis of life is the complex protein molecule round which the protoplasm of the living cell is built. These large molecules, with their branching side chains and interlocking configurations of simpler chemicals, contain essential elements called amino acids. The protein molecule attracts to itself from food-derived materials in the blood stream, those amino acids and other chemicals which it needs to keep itself in good repair and maintain its nourishment.

What would happen, asked Ehrlich, if the living protein molecule, reaching out for a suitable amino acid, accidentally grasped a poisonous chemical carried by a germ which had got into the blood? Damage to the cell inhabited by the living protein might result.

In order to rid itself of the harmful chemical, the human protein would try to sever the connecting link which it has made with the invader. But what if the invading germ makes its chemical 'bait' hang on tightly? (For, of course, germs are made of living protein molecules too and are interested in their own survival. To them, human cells are desirable residences.)

Ehrlich reasoned that the human molecule could break the connection with the foreigner at the next link. This would damage the cell somewhat, but not as badly as it would if the bacterial chemical remained connected. Cell proteins can repair themselves. So the human protein molecule sheds a link on one of its numerous side chains and the immediate threat is averted. But there are more germs about in the blood; so to protect itself, our human protein molecule starts manufacturing many replicas of the shed link and casting them off into the blood stream to fool the germs, which being programmed to seek out these links, pick them up under the impression that they are still keys which enable them to get into cells.

This is the simplified basis of Ehrlich's side-chain theory of immunity. It has stood the test of time and still forms one of the corner stones of the science of immunology. The shed, defensive links are called antibodies and the foreign protein which composes the germ is called the antigen (because it generates antibodies).

In Ehrlich's day, nobody had seen an antibody. Their presence was assumed by the side-chain theory which so neatly explained what happened when a person caught an infectious disease and developed immunity against it. Today, under the electronmicroscope, antigens and antibodies can be seen in close-up, and chemists have worked out their molecular structure down to the last atom, so we know that Ehrlich was right.

Let us look at the sequence of events when a person is infected with typhoid fever, a bacterial disease, one attack of which confers life-long immunity and against which protection can be given by inoculation with attenuated typhoid bacilli. After gaining entry to the body from contaminated food or water, the typhoid bacillus travels in the blood to the human cell, where the typhoid protein (antigen) attaches to a side chain on the human cell protein (antibody). The potentially cell-damaging antigen-antibody complex is shed and the cell is stimulated to make an excess of antibodies which are shed also as decoys for other typhoid bacilli which appear as the bacillus multiplies in the blood stream. If enough antibodies are produced to mop up most of the invaders, the patient will recover without serious illness. But, if the typhoid bacilli are too many, the defensive antibodies will be outnumbered and a clinical attack of typhoid fever will occur.

In this battle for immunity, typhoid bacilli which attach to human cells injure the latter, but things work both ways; cell-derived antibodies injure typhoid bacilli. Vaccination consists of injecting a small quantity of attenuated typhoid bacilli, well before the risk of catching typhoid occurs. This allows the body cells time to produce large quantities of floating antibody, so that if infection with typhoid occurs, the bacilli are destroyed before they have had time to multiply.

This antigen/antibody immune response is extraordinarily specific. A different antibody is produced to deal with each type of invader. Vaccination against smallpox virus is no protection at all against typhoid bacilli or the protozoal micro-organisms of sleeping sickness. And of course there are other defence mechanisms in the immune response besides the antigen/antibody reaction, some only recently discovered with more undoubtedly awaiting discovery, for immunology is constantly expanding. Phagocytosis was an early example first described in 1883 by Ilya Mechnikov (1845–1916) a Russian zoologist and bacteriologist who gave this name to the engulfment and digestion of bacteria and other foreign particles by white blood corpuscles. White cells, the scavengers of the blood stream, are greatly stimulated to eat up bacteria by the presence of antibodies, and it has been found that a coating of antibody on a bacterium makes it much more appetizing to the white cell phagocytes (from the Greek *phage* = eat and *cyt* = cell).

So intrigued did the intelligentsia become with the idea of phagocytosis and immunity in general, that George Bernard Shaw had one of the medical characters in his play *The Doctor's Dilemma* (1906) say practically nothing else but 'stimulate the phagocytes'. In those far-off days before the First World War doctors and patients really believed that science was winning the battle against disease. Unfortunately they were wrong.

In the feverish search for more science-based answers to the problems of infectious disease, in the hope that the vaccines developed against smallpox, rabies, typhoid and cholera would soon lead to a disease-free world, medical workers began to encounter some patients who reacted to the marvellous new treatments, not by becoming immune, but by suddenly dying.

So far in this brief history, we have been looking at prophylaxis (medical protection against disease, given in advance) in the context of immunization against the microbes causing contagious fevers. All seemed to be going well, when suddenly anaphylaxis (removal of protection), the evil twin sister of prophylaxis, appeared on the scene to terrify the medical investigators.

Inexplicably, some of their patients died as a direct result of further attempts to improve immunization. It started in the 1880s during the development of antitoxins.

The germs causing infectious diseases release toxins or poisons within the bodies of their hosts as they multiply and try to gain a foothold. Micro-organisms of diphtheria, tetanus and gas gangrene (the bane of men wounded in the trenches in the First World War) produce particularly virulent toxins which can damage the tissues of the body in various ways. During infection, the body of the host develops antitoxins which neutralize toxins, so it was a logical step for research workers to look for ways of producing antitoxin artificially in order to confer what is called passive immunity on people not already immunized who had already contracted, say, diphtheria or were in danger of doing so because of contact with a known case. For example, the anti-tetanus jab given routinely to people with dirty wounds in our hospital accident/emergency departments today is antitoxin.

This sort of protection was made available for the diphtheria contact or the person wounded on cultivated ground where tetanus was a risk, by means of injections of serum from horses containing diphtheria or tetanus antitoxin. It was with this procedure that unexpected deaths occurred. The sequence of events leading to this problem with serum-based antitoxin went as follows: Around 1887, Dr Henry Sewall, one of the first professors of physiology, was studying the action of rattlesnake venom at the University of Michigan at Ann Arbor. He would annoy his snakes and then slip a porcelain dish with a long handle down into the cage. The angry snakes would bite at the dish and deposit the venom from the tips of their hollow fangs. Sewall withdrew the dish and injected the venom into pigeons who died quickly.

He started giving them very small amounts, highly diluted, at frequent intervals and when he found that these small doses were not lethal, he gradually increased the dose until they could take the amount normally injected in a snake bite without untoward reaction. He had protected them.

This was not an entirely new idea. Early Greek history (100 BC) tells how Mithridates, King of Pontus (now part of Turkey), used to take small doses of various poisons daily in order to protect himself against a big dose which he feared an enemy might one day slip into his food. It worked, and he survived several attempts on his life with poison, only to die later by his own sword.

Learning of Sewall's work, Dr Albert Calmette at the Pasteur Institute in Paris showed that when the pigeons were injected with small doses of snake venom at frequent intervals an antitoxin was produced which he called antivenin. He and his team went on to inject horses with snake venom and found that they produced large quantities of antivenin in their blood. The blood was drawn off, allowed to clot and the clear serum containing the antitoxin, which separated was sterilized and sealed in glass tubes, ready for injection into victims of snake bites.

Calmette's horses were *actively* immunized and their blood continued to contain antivenin thereafter. People given antivenin in horse serum are *passively* immunized. Their cells are not stimulated to make more antivenin because they have not been confronted with the actual venom. The protection given by a shot of antivenin serum lasts about four weeks; long enough to get over a snake bite.

Next, Dr Pierre Roux, who had been Pasteur's assistant and later became Director of the Pasteur Institute, isolated the toxin produced by the diphtheria bacillus. He repeated Sewall's work, using diphtheria toxin instead of snake venom, and found that he could build up immunity to diphtheria toxin in animals.

Finally in 1890, Emil von Behring, a young German doctor, working under Roux, made a serum containing diphtheria antitoxin for passive immunization of children. This was a momentous advance. Diphtheria in the nineteenth century was as big a menace as smallpox had been in the eighteenth and there had been no cure. Doctors and parents had to sit helplessly by while children were slowly suffocated by the diphtheritic membrane which grew across their throats and blocked their air passages.

Von Behring read a paper on his discovery to the 1894 International Conference on Hygiene and Demography (population studies) in Budapest, attended by top European medical experts, on the epidemiology of infectious diseases. He told them how he had immunized horses against diphtheria toxin and then cured children of diphtheria by injecting them with the horse serum. There was a deadly silence; the scientists did not believe him. But when Pierre Roux told them he had checked von Behring's claims and found them true, the meeting of solemn, frock-coated doctors leapt to their feet clapping and cheering. It was the best news they had ever heard.

Dr von Behring gave them each an ampoule of his serum to try and the drug manufacturers started buying horses, growing diphtheria bacilli, extracting the toxin, injecting it into the horses, collecting and purifying the serum. Within a year, diphtheria antitoxin serum was being used on a wide scale by doctors throughout the civilized world.

In most cases it worked like magic, but before long disturbing reports of adverse reactions began to come in. Two of these came from America. In one case a doctor, who had been called to see a man with a sore throat and a raised temperature, found the tell-tale grey membrane and took a throat swab; the report came back: diphtheria bacilli had grown. Three minutes after the injection of diphtheria antitoxin in horse serum, the patient collapsed unconscious apparently about to die. The doctor, recognizing shock, gave several injections of adrenalin and just managed to save the man's life.

In another more tragic case, the doctor thought it a wise precaution to give prophylactic injections of antitoxin to other members of the family. The sick child's father who was well at the time dropped dead soon after receiving his injection. The condition was called serum sickness, but nobody knew the cause. In relation to the tens of thousands of people being immunized, there were not that many cases, but enough to worry doctors. So the search began to find out why. Which brings us into the twentieth century and the growing recognition of the importance of allergy.

Up to 1900, the medical profession had not recognized the basically similar pathology behind all those diverse diseases which we now call allergic. The word allergy had not been invented and although hay fever, asthma, urticaria, migraine and the rest had been described from earliest times, nobody suspected that there might be a connection between them.

The only available explanation for these strange maladies which seemed to be brought on in some people by contact with flowers, fur, feathers and drugs was idiosyncrasy (from the Greek: *idios* = own, *syn* = together and *krasis* = mixture). But this was just a descriptive label, meaning that the illness was peculiar to the patient's own constitution, not an explanation. Now, at last, with the coming recognition of serum sickness, a life-threatening reaction to something innocuous to most people, the key to the riddle was provided.

In 1901, Charles Richet, professor of physiology at the University of Paris, was studying toxins, as von Behring had done, but working on animals. He had started three years before, while cruising on Prince Albert of Monaco's yacht. The Prince was a keen scientist and oceanographer who liked men of Richet's calibre and Richet was glad of the opportunity to study the sting of the Portuguese man-of-war, a jelly fish of fearsome size, with trailing, stinging tentacles, which cause hives or urticaria when they touch skin.

Richet's work was not completed by the time he returned to Paris so he continued, using the sea-anemone instead of the

man-of-war. He made extracts of sea-anemone, injecting them
into dogs. When he gave large doses the dogs became ill; with
smaller doses they did not. Intermediate-size doses produced
symptoms of varying severity. He reasoned that if small doses
were harmless, he might be able to immunize the dogs against
larger doses by giving the weak injections at spaced intervals and
gradually increasing the dose until symptoms began to show,
thus conferring protection.

In the course of this work, something completely unexpected
happened which set Richet on a different course which was to
have far-reaching consequences for our understanding of allergy.

After the second or third weak injection, his dogs became very
ill. Something seemed to have happened to them in the interval
between injections, and the previously harmless material had
become highly poisonous in the same or even smaller doses than
those which had previously proved to be harmless.

Richet's colleague, Paul Portier, always the sceptic, asked to
watch one of these experiments. They chose a dog called Neptune,
a healthy animal, who three weeks previously had been given a very
small injection of sea-anemone extract which had not bothered
him. He was well when the two doctors examined him and gave
him a second injection. Neptune became violently ill and within
twenty-five minutes was dead. Dr Portier was impressed.

The discovery of this phenomenon, which Richet called
anaphylaxis (removal of protection) was the beginning of medical
understanding of allergy.[41] He thought that the substance which
induced anaphylaxis had to be toxic, but later found that non-
toxic substances such as blood serum would also induce anaphylaxis. The opposite term, prophylaxis meaning 'conferring
protection', had been used for a long time to describe vaccination
against smallpox, rabies and other infectious diseases.

In 1906, for the far more common, but usually less severe
clinical counterpart in man, von Pirquet suggested the word
'allergy' meaning a state of altered responses or reactivity.
Doerr[10], who was working with him, widened the use of the
word to cover all forms of altered reactivity, whether an underlying antigen/antibody reaction could be demonstrated or not.

This broad definition of allergy was later supported in the 1930s by Dr French K. Hansel, the founder of ear, nose and throat allergy in the USA, and other pioneers in food allergy in America: Albert Rowe, Arthur Coca, Warren T. Vaughan and Herbert Rinkel, and their pupils who went on to found the Society for Clinical Ecology.

At the same time, a rival school of immunological allergists was growing, which insisted on positive skin tests for the diagnosis of all kinds of allergy and used a massive build-up of antigen injections in the treatment of inhalant allergies to pollens, moulds and dusts. Because food allergens did not show up reliably with the type of skin test then in use, this school taught that food allergy was uncommon and tended to ignore it as a cause of their patient's symptoms. Thus came about the divergence of the two schools, based on a definite contribution to ignorance put about by the men who relied, and still do rely, exclusively on skin tests.

Quite rapidly, the study of clinical allergy came to be dominated by these doctors who used skin tests exclusively, followed by booster shots of the antigens to which patients had reacted with weals. They were able to corner the inhalant allergy market because of the prevalence of ragweed hay fever in the United States and because Leonard Noon at St Mary's Paddington had had wide publicity for his success in treating seasonal hay fever by injection of minute but increasing doses of pollen extract.[38]

By the late 1930s the majority of allergists had limited their activities to giving skin tests and shots for hay fever, asthma and urticaria, based on the antigen/antibody reaction theory. Anything which they could not explain and treat in these terms they pronounced 'not allergic'. As we shall see, this attitude – not unconnected with the high profit margin on shots – left a lot of patients dissatisfied.

Now to return to Richet and his anaphylaxis in the 1900s. At first he thought the injected material had to be slightly poisonous to produce the phenomenon. He was still thinking of toxins, but he wondered if completely non-irritating substances did likewise.

His colleague, Dr Maurice Arthus, found the answer to this question by looking for an organic substance which could not possibly be toxic. He decided that blood serum was the ideal substance. It could not be toxic, coursing as it did through the blood stream of all animals and coming into intimate contact with body cells and obviously essential to life. Arthus repeated Richet's experiments, substituting horse serum for sea-anemone extract and guinea pigs for dogs. Successive injections of serum, given not less than ten days apart, caused death from anaphylaxis.

This was a jolt for Richet's theory of removal of protection. You did not need protection against something as harmless as serum. Or did you? Richet knew von Pirquet, and von Pirquet, who was a paediatrician working on diphtheria antitoxin, had told him about serum sickness. Could anaphylaxis and serum sickness have the same cause? In 1905, von Pirquet and his associate, Dr Bela Schick, published their paper on serum sickness[40] giving their reasons for believing it to be a form of Richet's anaphylaxis. Not for the first time, the mystery of a lethal human disease looked like being solved by animal experiments in the physiology laboratory.

So, the most explosive form of allergy was the first to be studied experimentally in the laboratory. Even the challenge material used was the same both in humans and experimental animals: horse serum. In both cases the results could be deadly.

From this surprising finding and tie-up, it is easy to understand why hives or urticaria was soon suspected of being anaphylactic also, because most patients with serum sickness develop an urticarial rash. Asthma was the next 'idiosyncrasy' to be classed with anaphylaxis, because Arthus's guinea pigs wheezed before they died. Hay fever was soon suspect too but it took five more years before an explanation for anaphylaxis was formulated in terms of what was already known about immunity.

Richet received the coveted Nobel prize in 1913 for his work on anaphylaxis and ended his days, still the investigator, in a magnificent Louis XV mansion on the left bank of the Seine, studying the occult and visiting mediums, trying to procure a specimen of ectoplasm. In this he was not successful.

From his early work on immunity, Dr Victor Vaughan, the celebrated American allergist at Ann Arbor, Michigan, had concluded in 1907 that immunity and the newly christened disease, allergy (which included anaphylaxis), are different manifestations of the same fundamental response of body cells when confronted with bacteria or any other foreign protein. The idea was accepted readily by other investigators because, if true, it should explain allergy in terms of Ehrlich's well-established side-chain theory.

What would happen, asked Vaughan, if the mechanism for shedding antibody went wrong and instead of being cast off into the blood stream, the antibody remained firmly attached to the parent cell? There would not be enough free antibody to combine safely with all the invading foreign protein; and the foreign protein which locked on to the antibody still attached to the body cells might do damage. Much more recent immunological research has confirmed that this (with minor complications) is a fair account of what actually happens in allergy of the anaphylactic type. Why should the shedding of antibody go wrong? It is an old Army maxim that if it is possible for anything to go wrong, it will. Immunology is no exception.

We now know that all allergic reactions involve leakage of fluid from the tiny blood vessels into the tissues, causing swelling. The weals of urticaria or hives are an example of this kind of allergic swelling, affecting the skin.

The shock associated with anaphylaxis is due to massive loss of circulating fluid from the blood into the tissues. Hence the drip put up for shocked patients after accidents to run fluid quickly into a vein and make up the blood volume. Adrenalin constricts the smaller blood vessels and stops them from leaking.

That is really the end of the story of how allergy, the strangest malady of all, came to be explained by what generations of doctors and scientists have discovered about immunity to germs and to supposedly harmless serum proteins. One small problem remains: how can people become allergic to simple, non-protein chemicals like aspirin, nickel and chlorine?

When I was at medical school, a fellow-student was taken into hospital to have his tonsils out. After the operation, he told me how sore his throat felt and how the gargle the nurse was giving him did not seem to help. I had a packet of aspirin in my pocket, stirred them up in water in his drinking glass and told him to gargle and then swallow the stuff.

This was a remedy I found worked for me, when I had a sore throat, but to my horror, the effect was frightful. He developed asthma and went blue in the face, looking ready to suffocate. The Sister came bustling in, wanting to know what on earth was happening. When I told her, she gave me a withering ticking off and called the house surgeon who gave my colleague a shot of adrenalin, which put things right.

Richet had assumed that only proteins could cause anaphylaxis but other doctors began to point out that many quite simple drugs could do the same. Relatively simple foreign chemicals, like drugs, can combine with human serum proteins to turn them into antigens which could provoke cells to produce antibodies against them after absorption from the bowel. Such a drug or other chemical which combines with a protein to form a new, immunologically different protein, is called a hapten. In other words, a hapten cannot initiate an immune response, either favourable or unfavourable, unless attached to a protein carrier.

THREE

A case of chemical allergy?

All this preamble about how doctors and scientists began to understand immunity and its opposite, anaphylaxis or allergy, first to live, infectious micro-organisms and then to non-living substances in the environment, is necessary if we are to understand how more and more of us are becoming 'allergic to the twentieth century' to quote the phrase once used about himself by Professor William Rea. The predicament in which Dr Rea found himself in 1973 is a good example of how you or I or anyone else may become ill from exposure to chemicals in the environment, and how clinical ecology can come to the rescue.

Bill Rea is a fairly tall, thin man with a limp. His features are sharp; he has a long, thin nose and brown eyes and his quiet Texas drawl belies the brightness of his mind. 'Smart as a whip', an expression he used about a colleague, applies well to him but the overall impression one gets from talking to him is of uncompromising honesty and guts, laced with a fine, dry sense of humour. To hear him laugh, which he does often, is a tonic. Other things I noticed about him were his economy with words and time, his kindliness and his habit of ignoring non-essentials and getting straight to the point. He can, like Churchill could, 'switch off' at any time and go to sleep if he wants. He can also be very obstinate.

His wife is called Vera and they have four children of school age. They live in a biggish house on the outskirts of Dallas. I have seldom met a more united, charming and happy family. Two of the boys have quite severe food allergies but have learned to control them by avoiding certain foods and rotating the permitted ones. Like most American children I have met, their conversation is direct and uncompromising because they really do seem to want to know about people and things.

In 1970, Bill Rea's career as a successful cardiothoracic surgeon almost came to an end because of inexplicable attacks of dizziness and 'flu-like' symptoms which began to overcome him in the operating theatre. On one occasion he actually passed out. Things got so bad that he had to seek help, first from a general physician/allergist who gave him drugs which made him too dopey to work and secondly, from Dr Randolph in Chicago who diagnosed an ecological illness and set him on the road to a cure so that he was able to return to his exacting job.

He came to England in July 1978 to speak at a seminar on clinical ecology at the Basingstoke District Hospital Postgraduate Centre, and at a symposium on nutrition and social behaviour at the Royal Society of Medicine in London. While over here, he gave me an account of his illness and of how he got into clinical ecology.

R. M. Bill, would you tell me how you got started into clinical ecology?

W. R. Yes. About five years ago I got so dizzy I could not really stand up, and beginning to look into my problem I found out that I was allergic to many foods and it became evident that that was not the whole problem; about fifty per cent of it was due to chemicals and so I started reading about this, and read Rowe's book[49], and Rinkel and Randolph's book[47], and started attending the courses and just worked out the problem. My family also had it, they had been quite ill, my sons and my wife, and so that was extra evidence.

R. M. This was all working out your own problem, but when did you start to apply it to patients in the practice?

W. R. Probably six months to a year later. It became quite evident to me that many patients who were sent to me had manifestations of ecological disease and nobody was getting any help, or giving any help. So I started doing a few respiratory problems first, and then did some respiratory failures and then starting working on phlebitis, then vasculitis, then cardiac problems and then took on a whole gang of them after that.

R. M. But at that time you didn't have any unit; you must have been doing it in the ordinary wards?

W. R. Right, we did respiratory arrest patients and patients in the Intensive Care which was rather sound ecologically, and then when we put them out in the ward, we noticed they got worse, so we created one room out there for them and then as things grew, then we went to two rooms and then three and then four and things got so cumbersome with four rooms that the hospital thought we ought to have a wing so we started the wing. We did this probably over a period of two years.

R. M. So what year would this bring us up to?

W. R. 1975.

R. M. Could you tell me about the mortician you mentioned. He sounded a good case.

W. R. Yes. He was thirty-seven years old, had been a mortician all his life and his father before him. He had hardening of the arteries and heart pain. They did a bypass on him because they found on coronary angiogram that he did have narrowing of the coronary arteries. But he went on having chest pain and arrhythmia.

R. M. When did he have the bypass?

W. R. About two years ago.

R. M. How soon did he come to you after that?

W. R. About a year after the bypass he came. We placed him in the unit, fasted him, and took him off all his medicines and in five days he was totally clear and we went ahead and challenged him on beef which reproduced all his symptoms. And I think, one other food. His challenge with formaldehyde also reproduced it and when the story came out that as a child he slept over the embalming area all his life, so he apparently had plenty of years of sensitizing substance.

R. M. Did he have any other chemical allergies besides formaldehyde?

W. R. I think chlorine bothered him also, because he was having a swimming pool built with chlorine and decided to change that. He was getting that fixed for rehabilitation for his heart.

R. M. And the interest in ecology really sprang from having felt unwell yourself in the theatre? Do you think this was triggered by the anaesthetics?

W. R.   Yes, definitely it was. Anaesthetics and the fumes of the heart/lung machine, both of these things. I would go in when I was in training in thoracic surgery, on a Monday and leave on Saturday morning. You know, you've got that machine all the time and all that anaesthetic all the time.

R. M.   What are the specific chemicals they have coming at you from those machines?

W. R.   Well, the machines have just motor exhausts and there are a lot of plastics around and then the anaesthetic, a lot of that nitrous oxide and flurothane, chlorinated hydrocarbons, in other words.

R. M.   So that really triggered it. But did you get any warning before this particular attack, did you have smaller ones?

W. R.   Oh yes, I used to get headaches and they got gradually worse. They were vascular type and I would get periods of fatigue and a lot of muscle aches and irritable colon and then I got sore throats, all the time and flu-like symptoms, and before I really discovered what it was, my wife made the statement, 'Nobody can have flu 365 days out of a year.' Recurrent sinus all the time ... you know.

R. M.   When did it actually come to the point where you had treatment? Did you go and see Randolph or did you do it for yourself?

W. R.   No, the first thing in 1970, I did go to see a classical allergist, he started me on shots which did not help and gave me drugs. The more drugs I took the worse I got, until he had me on about twelve pills a day, of different things and I couldn't see straight – ridiculous – you know. And then I got to talking to this former medical student of mine and he said, 'You have got food allergy.'

R. M.   Now how did he know?

W. R.   Because he's had it.

R. M.   He learned about it from Randolph?

W. R.   Yes, indirectly, it was some of the guys who had taken the course, some ENT guys got him on to it.

R. M. Was he a patient himself?

W. R. Yes, he had been a patient with them and I went out to his office and did some skin testing and it became quite evident to me that it was much deeper than that.

R. M. This was Joe Miller's skin testing?[36]

W. R. Yes.

R. M. Did you go to see Joe?

W. R. No, I didn't know about Joe at the time.

R. M. And have you always used his methods and had these bottles for doing it? (*The bottles were his food and chemical extracts which he took with him when travelling, to keep himself immunized.*)

R. M. So now, how do you keep yourself well, because you have a very hard life, you work long hours.

W. R. I have a good home, it's ecologically sound, good office and a good unit. The operating rooms are pretty good now and I never wear clothes that aren't all cotton, and aren't all washable, and I rarely eat out.

R. M. I have seen your kitchen with a big extractor over the range. No gas, everything electric.

W. R. I just really try to take care of myself very well and when we travel we take our own water and then some food and we really manage very well.

R. M. How much do you use shots to turn yourself off?

W. R. Well, I take food shots and also pollen, dust and mould shots and terpenes.*

R. M. All the time?

W. R. Every four days.

R. M. Every four days you give yourself terpenes, mould, dust, pollen and how many foods?

W. R. Sixty.

---

*Terpenes are responsible for the odour and taste of plants. There are more terpenes in the world than any other plant products. Resins are terpenes, so is the latex of the rubber tree. They have been called nature's petrochemicals and give rise to our oil, coal and gas deposits and fossil fuels. Immunization against terpenes can protect against allergy to domestic gas and motor car fumes.

R. M.   And you still rotate your diet?

W. R.   Always, we always rotate it.

R. M.   That's on a four-day rotation?

W. R.   Oh, it's more like two weeks.

R. M.   Two weeks' rotation, and you eat once a day?

W. R.   Yes, although we have been breaking that over here recently, sometimes we eat twice but at home I only eat once a day.

R. M.   And how many foods do you eat at a time?

W. R.   Oh, two or three, sometimes four.

R. M.   And you have got enough foods to do a fortnight's rotation?

W. R.   Some of those foods, even longer.

R. M.   And on that you keep really well?

W. R.   Well, I keep so I work eighteen hours a day, I wouldn't say I am really well, but . . .

R. M.   Well you look alright!

W. R.   I am not what I want to be, put it that way.

I have deliberately given this interview with Professor Rea to show how all our hard-won understanding of allergic people and processes can be put to practical use. The basics were known by 1912 so a jump to a real case in 1978 shows how relevant the early work still is.

Bill Rea has found ways of protecting himself. Of course, many more details are now known about what goes on inside the body in health and disease, but when you get ill, you can still only do so in eight different ways. Here are the diagnostic choices open to you or your doctor, if you find yourself in some sort of trouble; you can:

1 be born with a defect

2 be injured

3 start wearing out

4 catch an infection and suffer the effects of not overcoming it completely

5 develop a tumour or new growth, which may or may not be spreading and invading other tissues

6   fail to adapt to something in your environment which does
not seem to bother other people (become allergic)
7   suffer some sort of poisoning or
8   become upset psychologically by interaction with another
person or life situation.

As a doctor, Rea knew all this and the possibilities must have
gone rapidly through his mind when he became ill. If he had had
an inborn defect it would have shown up before his forties. He
was too young to be wearing out. So was it an infection? His
wife Vera put down that idea when she said: 'Nobody can have
flu 365 days out of a year', by which she meant that flu gives
you a short attack which confers some temporary immunity.
You may catch another doss of flu later caused by a different
virus, but flu symptoms do not go on reappearing day after day
for a year. Had he got cancer? Maybe. Cancer can be a great
mimic but it does not usually present with so many alternating
symptoms. It usually starts silently and then gradually and
steadily produces a mounting level of aches, pains and other things
going wrong.

So he considered allergy and went to the nearest allergist, an
orthodox man who had only two approaches: skin tests followed
by shots of anything which reacted on the skin, and when that
did not work, drugs to suppress symptoms. Even on twelve pills
a day, he only felt worse.

Then he was lucky. He ran into a former medical student of
his who had had a similar illness and knew it to be caused by food
allergy. Nearly every doctor in the field of clinical ecology has,
or has had, an allergic illness himself or in his immediate family.
They can tell stories like Bill Rea's. I know I can. Had I not met
Dr Randolph by a lucky chance in 1958, I might still be flounder-
ing around looking for a cure for the intermittent fatigue, depression and irritable colon which used to afflict me.

Adaptive breakdown does not show itself in any two people
in exactly the same way. We are all individuals. Our finger prints
are all different so it is not surprising that within an overall
similar pattern, your biochemistry is unique to you and different

from mine and therefore your responses to allergenic substances will be peculiar to yourself.

We saw how the guinea pig developed severe wheezing in anaphylaxis. Plenty of allergic humans do the same in an allergic reaction. Your particular target organ could be your muscles or your joints. If allergy can affect your lungs or your heart, why not your brain? Of the 400,000 hospital beds in the NHS nearly half are occupied by mental patients.

How many of these people are ill because their brains are the target of allergic reactions to certain foods, drugs or chemicals in the air? I have treated scores of them and suspect that as many as one in every three patients going to GPs and psychiatrists with so-called emotional problems are really allergic. If I am right then psychiatry is due for a drastic shake up.

So here you are, stuck perhaps with one of the three most common diagnostic labels today: high blood pressure, bowel disorder or an emotional (behavioural) problem, or maybe just feeling sick and tired all over. You have seen the specialist, several even, and they have handed you back to your GP with a prescription for drugs and a sheaf of negative special investigations. Where do you go? What do you do?

The *Worthing Gazette* headlined an article 'Why life without plastic is bliss for Pat'[57]. Mrs Pat Berney was photographed sitting beside, and giving the thumbs down sign to the gas-fired wall-fitted water heater, several plastic containers for various domestic liquids and a plastic curtain. She and her husband Derek used to run a pub in the village of Amberley and an incident involving the plastic drip trays under the beer taps finally decided them both to call 'time' and start living more as nature intended.

Nearly all her life, Pat had had many mysterious illnesses with pain, swelling, sickness, headaches and blackouts until she thought she was going crazy. She even had convulsions after eating certain foods. Then one day when drawing a pint of beer she blacked out and sent the beer flying over a customer. When she came round she remembered that just before pulling the pint of beer she had been washing the plastic drip trays, and conversations she had

had with the organizer of the local Allergy Group made her suspect that she might have had a reaction to the plastic drip trays. She consulted a doctor who specialized in clinical ecology and as a result she and her husband bought an all-electric cottage which was stripped of all things plastic, and in which Pat found she could live without too many symptoms.

Said Pat, 'Finding the Allergy Group here has helped me enormously because I know I am not going mad and I no longer feel alone because there are plenty of other people in the same boat. I think I am lucky to have found out the cause of my mysterious illness and I am now trying to help others in the group.'

Your problem may be the same as Professor Rea's. So let us look at his story again and try to see what guidance can be obtained. He proved that the fumes from the anaesthetic gases and the heart/lung machine had sensitized him to petrochemicals – so he de-sensitizes himself with an injection of terpene extracts every four days, which enables him to work in the presence of these fumes without getting a headache or feeling dizzy. His pollen, mould and dust allergies are controlled in the same way. His food allergies have been worked out, so he excludes his worst offenders and takes shots to boost his immunity to those he cannot avoid. He rotates his permitted foods through a two week cycle so as not to create new allergies by eating and drinking the same things day after day. All his foods are organically produced to avoid swallowing chemicals added on the farm or during processing and his home and office are as free of polluting chemicals, odorous plastics, moth-proofing, oil-burning appliances, etc. as it is possible to make them.

For the person only mildly allergic to foods and chemicals, a less rigorous programme may suffice, but if you have as many allergies as he does, you will have to be prepared to go to similar lengths to get well.

To illustrate the point, I give the following case. Some years ago I was asked to see a man on one of the psychiatric wards who, besides the depression for which he had been admitted, complained of pains in the back on his neck and inability to turn his head more than a few degrees to either side. He was a heavy smoker and I persuaded him to give up smoking for two weeks and to spend as much time as possible out of doors in the fresh air. After ten days his pain had gone and he could bring his chin round over either shoulder.

To challenge him with tobacco, I took one of his own cigarettes, lit it and blew the smoke repeatedly down a glass tube into a little distilled water in a cup. When he was sitting comfortably in an easy chair, without any pain in his neck, I placed two drops of the cigarette smoke solution under his tongue and told him to hold it there without swallowing. All was well for about a minute. Then suddenly he was convulsed with pain, crouching down in the chair and bringing his hands up to support his head. Asked to describe the pain, he said it felt like a four inch nail being driven down the back of his neck. The pain gradually eased off when progressively more dilute drops of the tobacco smoke solution were placed under his tongue. It was not difficult after this to persuade him to give up smoking altogether.

A lot of measures can be taken without medical help (avoidance manoeuvres) and these will be described as we go along. You will need the help of a doctor who practises clinical ecology if neutralization of allergens or de-sensitization is required. At present there are not many such doctors but with the growth of clinical ecology as a subject within medicine now taking place rapidly, my hope is that this kind of help will be available from GPs and hospitals in most areas before long.

FOUR

Chemical adulteration of food

Nearly thirty years ago, in 1951, in his opening address to the conference on *Problems Arising from the Use of Chemicals in Food*[48] held in London, Dr G. Roche Lynch, Home Office pathologist and toxicologist and a world authority on forensic medicine, said, 'When one peruses the formidable list of substances embraced by this conference, one is struck by the fact that, however necessary these substances are today, not one of them is of the slightest value to the nutrition of the human organism. The corollary of this is: to what extent may these substances be harmful?' He went on ... 'We know so little about many food additives, and what we do know tends to raise one's doubts rather than allay them.'

Eighteen years later, the *Lancet* in an editorial on food additives[25] wrote, 'The question of the ultimate effect of food additives on man is still unanswered.' Now, in 1979, the question becomes more urgent as the quantities and diversity of synthetic chemicals put into food mount while any claim that their safety is monitored in ways relevant to human health is being seriously questioned.

In 1950 the American Congress had already considered the problem of chemical additives in the food supply. In that year, the House of Representatives took evidence from dozens of expert witnesses testifying against the addition to food of new substances which were inadequately tested, sometimes hazardous and frequently unnecessary. The taking of this evidence, known as the Delaney Hearings, after the chairman, James T. Delaney, went on until 1958 and culminated in an amendment to the Original Food, Drug and Cosmetic Act of 1938, requiring pretesting of additives (on animals). Within two years of this amendment, the Food and Drugs administration had received

391 petitions for additional regulations concerning 1,900 uses
of chemicals in food production, processing and handling.

The 1960s saw an enormous rise in the production and consumption of *convenience* foods which depend on a host of
chemical stabilizers, flavourants, extenders, colours, preservatives
and antioxidants to keep them acceptable and marketable during
storage, handling, transport, freezing and reheating over a long
period of time. More hearings on chemical problems came and
various congressional committees were set up to investigate food
dyes, additives in sweets and pesticide residues in food. But they
were looking at the tip of the iceberg.

By 1970 the number of food additives covered by formal
regulations had risen to 2,703 and still the applications poured in.
A number of chemicals not covered by regulations were put on
the GRAS list (Generally Regarded As Safe) pending any report
coming in about harmful effects. Sheer numbers precluded
official testing of all but a few. Meanwhile, sales of additives to
food processors in the United States boomed.

In the early 1970s, sales of chemical additives to food proces-
sers amounted to $500 million annually. The figure for 1980 is
expected to top $750 million. And what did all the testing amount
to ? It could not be done on humans, so rats, mice and guinea pigs
were mostly used, animals which are cheap, require little space
and breed well under laboratory conditions. But, the physiology
of a rat differs from that of a human in many respects. For in-
stance the widely used antioxidant, butylated hydroxytoluene, is
metabolized and excreted by different pathways in the human.
A disease resembling ulcerative colitis can be produced in the
guinea pig by carrageenan, a vegetable gum widely used in the
food industry, which appears not to have this effect in humans.

Safety regulations on additives are based on acute and chronic
toxicity studies in animals, i.e. how many animals in a batch
will the chemical kill. Toxicologists subject the animals to the
LD50 test to find the lethal (L) dose (D) for fifty per cent of the
animals in the test group so the lower the LD dose, the greater
the toxicity. If the LD50 is below 1 mg per kg of body weight,
the substance being tested is judged to be 'of extreme toxicity'.

Between 50 and 500 mg/kg is 'of moderate toxicity' and above 500 mg/kg 'of low toxicity'. Such information is valuable for drugs, which are mainly used singly, but not so valuable with food additives (chemicals), which are eaten combined with foods and other additives, day after day, year after year.

In fact the application of techniques for testing for drug safety to testing food additives is inappropriate. Sub-acute and chronic testing of additives gives more information, but is costly and time-consuming. In sub-acute toxicity tests, animals are given the additive for ninety days, during which blood and urine samples are taken. The animals are then killed and thirty different tissues examined microscopically for damage – kidneys, liver and spleen often show evidence of harm, none of which is necessarily relevant to subtle changes in human biological systems.

In a chronic toxicity test, an additive is put into a test animal's diet for its lifespan (two years in the rat). Some animals are sacrificed and their organs examined at six months and one year. Others are allowed to go on until they die. Such tests give information on growth rate, appetite, behaviour, life span and a number of biochemical and blood variables.

Although it is true that sub-acute and chronic toxicity tests give far more information than acute LD50 tests, they still have limited value for human protection. If an additive produces no observable damage from chronic toxicity studies, a 'no effect' level is established and the chemical is allowed to be put into food.

But these studies only look for observable injury to a range of organs in animals, far removed from man in structure and function. The establishment of a no-effect level for an additive does not ensure its safety, because no-effect levels *had* been shown in several additives which subsequently came to be banned.

What are food additives? They are chemical substances used to improve the keeping qualities, taste, texture and colour of manufactured foods and drinks. Other chemical additives, facilitate mechanical methods of food production and are best described as processing aids. Not all additives, as so defined, are harmful: common salt, added to dough in breadmaking to improve flavour, has been used since Biblical times without ill effect.

Contaminants, on the other hand, are not introduced deliberately into food and may be positively harmful, even dangerous. To supply food in abundance to townspeople at a reasonable price, farmers have to protect animals and crops from pests and use growth-promoting hormones and biocides in order to increase yield and reduce losses during production, harvesting, storage and distribution. Residues of a wide range of contaminating chemicals get into food in this way and others may be picked up accidentally from the environment. Heavy metals, such as lead and mercury, may accumulate in plants and animals near smelting plants and road junctions, or in fish in water polluted with factory effluent. Mineral oil may contaminate food processed and moved by machinery and plastic wrapping and tin can linings may be leached into foods and drinks during storage.

The amounts of additives and contaminants in food are seldom great enough to be toxic, although their long-term effects are unknown. But they are present in amounts well within the allergy-causing range in susceptible people.

Toxicity studies are not tackling the danger from allergy to chemical additives. The tests may protect us to some extent but do nothing to tell us whether we may become allergic or react adversely in other subtle ways peculiar to whole human beings.

As Dr Randolph pointed out[44]: 'Our analytical investigators seem to have wandered away from the question they set out to solve; the more minutely they subdivide the problem, the more difficult it is to rejoin its parts ... the sum of the toxicologist's analytical data is far removed from the situation confronting humans in their daily lives.'

In 1948 Dr Stephen Lockey[29], chief of the Department of Allergy of Lancaster General Hospital, Lancaster, Pennsylvania, published his first paper on allergy to dyes used to colour and identify various pills and tablets. He has gone on to publish many articles on colouring agents, flavourants and preservatives in foods and medicines to which people can have sensitivity reactions.

One case among many which Dr Lockey has described was a fifty-three year-old male whose doctor had prescribed a sedative: elixir of phenobarbitol (coloured with the F. D. & C. red dye known also as amaranth). Each time this patient took a tea-spoonful of the elixir he would rapidly develop generalized itching and urticaria with swelling of his lips, tongue and uvula which threatened to asphyxiate him. One quarter grain sodium pheno-barbitone tablet (uncoloured) had no ill effect, but sublingual challenge with 1 millilitre of Number 2 dilution of amaranth F. D. & C. red (containing 2 mg of dye) precipitated itching and swelling within a few minutes. The dilutions of dye were made with triple distilled, de-ionized water and the method of testing was as follows:

1 Patient was blindfolded.

2 One millilitre of Number 2 dilution placed under the tongue.

3 Patient observed for 20 minutes for signs of reaction.

4 If no reaction to dilution Number 2, patient was re-tested with dilution Number 1, containing 20 mg of the dye.

5 In making dilutions and testing, a standard, calibrated glass pipette and medicine dropper were used.

6 To avoid possible cumulative effects, not more than 2 dilutions of any primary F. D. & C. dye were tested per day.

Amaranth red is used to colour many foods, toiletries and medi-cines including gelatin-based toppings, maraschino cherries, sausage casings, carbonated drinks, dry drink powders, con-fectionary, soaps, ointments, suntan oils, tablets, capsules and mouthwashes.

Toxicity studies on animals have cleared many of the chemical additives in bread as 'safe' for human consumption, but the irrelevance of these animal tests to the well-being of some humans fed on modern bread is well illustrated by the case of a boy who came under my care some years ago.

Since the age of thirteen, James, who was an only child, had suffered from uncontrollable twitchings of his face, head and neck. When they were very bad, they involved his whole body, giving the impression of a puppet being jerked by its strings.

They stopped only when he was asleep. He had been taken to several specialists. A neurologist had investigated him thoroughly as an in-patient. Nothing had been found to account for his affliction and eventually at the age of sixteen, after disrupted schooling and rejection by everyone except his parents, he was sent to Basingstoke as a psychiatric case.

Every drug for the control of muscular spasm had been tried and, when he was first put under me, he was heavily addicted to a sleeping pill which he had been allowed to take by day and by night and was on a load of tranquillizers besides. He was also chain-smoking cigarettes. He was a very depressed, disturbed boy and his parents were at their wit's end as to what to do with him.

The year before he came to me, I had had a gratifying success with a disturbed and suicidal young woman who had lost all her symptoms on a five-day fast, and had subsequently done well on a diet which excluded all those items which had been shown to bring her symptoms back on double-blind tube feeding.* I was encouraged as a result of this case to try the technique on other seemingly hopeless cases.

James was put on a total fast with nothing but water to drink and his load of drugs and tobacco reduced. By the end of the fast his twitch had gone. On challenge with drops under his tongue of watery solutions of the foods he had been eating regularly in the past, only two brought back his twitch; white flour and yeast. The nurses and I found this surprising, until I saw from his notes that his father was a master baker and James had lived all his life over the bakery, inhaling the dust containing flour and yeast particles (remember Dr Rea's case of the mortician who became allergic to the formaldehyde in his father's embalming area).

On a diet which omitted all foods derived from wheat and other cereal grains and all foods and drinks containing yeast, James remained well, relapsing only when he broke his diet.

*A statistically controlled randomized study, done under controlled conditions in which neither the test subject nor the investigator is aware of the nature of the regimen.

Told baldly like this, his story sounds almost too pat and simple and of course his final rehabilitation was not simple at all and took two more years.

First the other doctors had to be convinced that a cause for his twitching had been found. James had been seen several times at our weekly case conferences and everybody knew him. I showed him again and he was so apprehensive that he trembled quite noticeably throughout the half hour he spent being questioned by the doctors, students and social workers present. Sceptical doctors suggested that he was really not much better and that the improvement was coincidental. Only time would answer this and it was decided to review his case again after six months. In fact his trembling at the meeting was quite unlike his spasmodic twitch.

Secondly, he had to be weaned off his drugs and cigarettes. I had reduced them but he was convinced that he still needed them. That took a long time, but eventually he gave them all up and seemed better for it.

Thirdly, there was the problem of his education and future. All this time I had kept him in hospital because returning home to the bakery brought back his twitch acutely. There were arguments with his parents who, quite rightly, were concerned about all the education he had missed and his job prospects. The only work he had ever done was helping on the bread delivery round from his father's van – not a suitable job for an intelligent twenty year old with ambitions to be a journalist.

Over the education, we had a stroke of luck. I telephoned the local Chief Education Officer, who turned out to be a marvellous man. He came to the hospital and interviewed James several times with and without me. The upshot was a student's grant, and a place at technical college to study for the 'O' levels and 'A' levels he had missed. James worked hard, coming top in his classes and passing all his exams first time. Socially he became a success, being elected president of his student's union. He developed a fine line in ironic repartee and during his vacations worked as a group leader at a youth club where he put on plays and projects with the teenagers in his charge. He won a place at university to read English and is currently working happily on a local newspaper as a trainee reporter.

The advent of the Chief Education Officer on the scene at a critical point in James's recovery underlines something which has again and again bolstered my faith in human nature. When everything seems to be getting difficult, suddenly you meet someone who is not obstructive, not insensitive, not bigoted but goodhearted and open-minded. Solution of your problem seems possible once more. So it was with James and so it has been at other points in my life when I have felt discouraged.

James's case illustrates another point, more immediately relevant to the theme of this book: the need for the logical scientific approach to every patient suspected of having an ecological illness.

Conclusions drawn from the results of the case: an abnormal or allergic reaction to some things in flour and yeast was upsetting the part of his brain concerned with posture and muscular movement. This could be an ecological or environmentally-triggered disease, and the implication was that similar symptoms involving the nervous system in other patients might have this same cause.

I have returned to the scientific, experimental approach with James because just at the time when I appeared to have solved his problem, I was given an opportunity to study him and three other ecological patients more intensively in a laboratory under controlled conditions.

Fisons, the big British firm of agricultural chemists, has a pharmaceutical division which for more than ten years has marketed a product called Intal, for the prevention of allergic asthma. It consists of powdered sodium cromoglycate, a substance found to have the unusual property of stabilizing the cells of the animal and human immunity systems (i.e. the so-called mast cells concerned in the antigen/antibody reaction to foreign substances, explained on page 33). By taking Intal into the lungs, via a special inhaler, *before* going outdoors and meeting the pollen which causes allergic wheezing, the asthma subject can protect himself. The Intal will prevent the cellular explosion and release of vaso-active histamine and other irritating substances into the blood stream when pollen antigen latches on to the cell-attached antibody in the lungs, so the asthmatic attack will not occur.

The set-up at Fisons laboratory consisted of an adjustable X-ray-type couch on which the subject of the experiment lay, connected by electrical leads to a console behind which a battery of pens drew lines on a moving strip of paper. Each pen recorded a different parameter e.g. pulse rate, respiration, temperature, electro-encephalogram (EEG or brain waves), electro-cardiogram (ECG or electrical potentials from heart muscle), electrical resistance of skin, etc.

The idea was to get basic recordings of all these things and then challenge the subject with drops under the tongue of a food to which he was known to be allergic and had avoided, with or without protective drops of Intal first. It was hoped that an allergic reaction would show up in alterations in the tracings made by the pens and that we could find out whether Intal had a protective action or not. To rule out any bias or psychological effect, the whole experiment was done double-blind; with real Intal drops, dummy Intal drops, white flour, and another food (soya) to which tolerance had been demonstrated in all four patients. All solutions came in coded, capped bottles, made up in Fisons pharmacy and no one involved in the experiment knew which was which.

The sequence of test was as follows:

1 Subject kept solution under the tongue for two minutes (time to block off the allergy cell receptors).

2 Mouth rinsed with distilled water.

3 Recording pens started writing, paper running.

4 Challenge with two drops of flour or soya solution (nobody knew which).

5 Tracing paper continued to run for two minutes (time to absorb the allergen).

6 Everything switched off, mouth rinsed again. Subject disconnected from the electrical leads.

All four patients were tested with every possible combination and the whole experiment took a week. It required a lot of patience and at times I nearly went to sleep. In one of my moments of inattention I missed seeing James give an involuntary twitch of his right arm soon after a food drop challenge went under his tongue. But the other doctor there saw it and so did the technician working the console and the paper tracings of the moving pens. With some of the challenges on the other three patients, the pens seem to go completely haywire, running right off the paper in one or two instances.

When we broke the code at the end of the week in the Medical Director's office, there was some jubilation because the wheat flour *had* produced violent changes in some of the tracings, while the soya had not and the Intal had had a protective effect.

So what had we proved? In James's case, that white flour in minute dosage, introduced into his blood stream via the veins close to the surface of the floor of his mouth, would make him twitch and in him and the three other people tested, challenge with white flour would induce changes in functions such as pulse, ECG and EEG over which they had no conscious control.

Intal (sodium cromoglycate is the active constituent) had been shown to exert a blocking action on these allergic responses which gave Fisons additional evidence to back their claim that the stuff had a protective effect against food allergy, as well as against inhalent allergens. Eventually, they put it on the market as Nalcrom, in capsules to be swallowed before food to enable some food-allergic people to eat things again which they had learned to avoid in order to keep well. It certainly works for some people, me included. I carry a few capsules and swallow them if I have to eat out. But it does not work for everyone with food allergy and some patients who have used it continuously have found the good effect wearing off after a year or more.

There seems to me to be a sort of justice in this endeavour of Fisons to find an antidote to food allergy, since their agricultural division sells to farmers some of the chemicals which can cause allergy in susceptible people. As most farmers are not likely to work without chemicals, it seems right that the chemical manu-

facturers should be looking for antidotes to allergy. The same
co-operation from the food manufacturers would go a long way
towards solving other growing ecological problems.

It would have been logical to challenge James with the chemical
additives his father put into the bread one at a time to see if any
brought back his twitch. James did bring me six test tubes full of
different chemicals his father used, but by that time he was well
and keen to get away from the hospital and all the bad associations
it had for him so they were never done. However, I have tested
stoneground wholemeal flour on other patients with allergy to
white flour and found that they could tolerate it. So the chemical
manipulation and treatment that flour undergoes when being
made into modern white bread, may render it more allergenic.
To look at it and taste it you would think so.

It is worth noting just what does go into a gummy supermarket
sliced white loaf:

Typical formula for commercial white bread.[16]

Ingredients

Enriched all-purpose flour	45 kg (100 lb)
Yeast	700–1150g (1½–2½ lb)
Enzyme-active soyaflour preparation	450 g (1 lb)
Salt	900 g (2 lb)
Sugar	1500 g (3 lb)
Lard	900–1500 g (2–3 lb)
Skim milk powder	900 g (2 lb)
Mono and di-glycerides	140 g (5 oz)
Calcium propionate	75–100 g (3–4 oz)

Additives (per cent)

Carrier (wheat starch)	0.0230
Bleach: benzoyl peroxide	0.0066
Free-flowing agents:	
tricalcium phosphate	0.0016
magnesium carbonate	0.00006
Maturing agent:	
potassium bromate	0.0011

Enrichment
  Iron   0.0027
B Vitamins
  Niacin   0.0030
  Thiamine mononitrate   0.0004
  Riboflavin   0.0003

Total additives (per cent)   0.03876

                                                             ozs
Yeast food   4–8

Composition (per cent)
  White flour   40.0
  Salt   25.0
  Calcium sulphate   25.0
  Ammonium chloride   9.7
  Potassium bromate   0.3

If we examine this formula more closely, some worrying things
emerge for the potentially allergic person or anyone concerned
about long-term toxicity or nutritional value for money. Enzyme-
active soya flour preparation contains lipoxidase to further bleach
the flour and improve dough mixing and flavour. It also contains
pre-gelatinized cornstarch which can affect anyone allergic to
corn. Skim milk powder is put in too, and can be a hazard
to anyone with a cow's milk allergy who does not know it is
there.

Although the dough formula contains adequate sugar and
minerals for the growth of yeast, bakers have long added extra
'yeast food' to aid what they call a smooth fermentation. This is
really a device for blowing up the bread with more air and thus
giving more bread for less dough; potassium bromate is an oxidiz-
ing agent which keeps air in the dough while it bakes and stiffens
the protein molecules. It is not necessary for feeding the yeast.
Some years ago, this practice resulted in such monstrously
inflated bread that one pound loaves ended up the size and shape
of one-and-a-half pound loaves. In Oregon, in 1964, this de-

ception was countered with legislation that such bread be labelled as 'balloon bread'.

Notice that three to four ounces of calcium propionate are included. Propionates are mould retarding agents which make the bread 'stay fresh longer'; manifestly a contradiction in terms. Good bread should go stale. These fungicidal anti-enzymes destroy the vital processes which enable moulds and fungi to grow and breed. They are also common ingredients in ointments for treating fungal infections of the skin like athletes' foot. Calcium propionate inhibits the enzyme which enables the human body to assimilate calcium – a serious matter for growing children and pregnant women.

It may be reassuring to learn that propionates are naturally present in cheeses but less so when cheese is known to be one of the most commonly incriminated foods in migraine and other allergic illnesses. Gastro-intestinal allergy has been reported four to eighteen hours after eating foods containing propionates.[55]

Mono- and di-glycerides are described by the industry as softeners, besides being anti-staling agents and volume improvers. They enter the starch granule, preventing it from setting up a rigid matrix by reaction with water and thus going hard and stale. What all this means in terms of nutrition is not known, because long ago the baking industry chose to symbolize food value in terms of softness, smoothness and whiteness. Public revolt against these totally irrelevant criteria, as expressed in the couplet 'the whiter the bread, the sooner you're dead!' has recently led to emphasis on enrichment and home-baked qualities in advertisements for factory-produced bread. The three vitamins included in the commercial formula I have quoted do not enrich flour but merely restore partially the massive vitamin depletion which occurs during manufacture.

As we move into the 1980s, less and less of our money goes on real food – more and more on processing, artificial ingredients, chemical preservatives, packaging, advertising and display. Study of any highly processed food – especially one with a high promotional budget – shows it to be far more costly than its basic food ingredients. The cost of a dry breakfast cereal, for example, is many times more than the cost of the grains from which it is manufactured. Part of the cost of any processed food goes on advertising and a lot more on stopping perishable basic carbohydrates, fats and proteins from going bad by freezing, dehydrating, homogenizing, condensing and vacuum packing after stabilizing their constituent molecules with anti-staling chemical agents.

For the allergic patient the safest kinds of processed food are quick-frozen fruit, vegetables and fish, because they do not contain chemical preservatives. It is possible for peas and some other crops, which are gathered mechanically in bulk, to be affected by spray residues but, as a general rule, I have found patients better able to tolerate quick-frozen vegetables rather than canned.

Every day, 'new' food items are displayed on supermarket shelves but over the last hundred years total food consumption in weight-conscious Western countries has gone down, resulting in ever fiercer competition among the food manufacturers for a corner in that shrinking 1.10 kg container, the human stomach.

There is now a battle being waged in every supermarket in the land for space in your stomach and intestines.

In 1900 a grocer's shop would sell less than one hundred items, mainly raised on nearby farms and eaten at once after home preparation or storage in dried or bottled form. Today, the average supermarket stocks around 8,000 different items.

The food purveyor is no longer concerned with selling quality but with display; there is a battle between producers for shelf space at eye level, resulting in 'hidden' bribes such as gifts, coupons and stickers. The customer is attracted by 'giant', 'jumbo' and 'kingsize' in the same way.

Contrary to popular mythology about the hard-headed male sex, men out shopping are more susceptible to this sales gimmickry than women. They are suckers for pleasant lighting, free snacks, chocolate-aroma aerosols and muzak, the all-pervading background music.

Clinical ecologists believe that the enormous leap in the number of sufferers from chemical allergy is a side effect of the switch from honest trading of good food to reliance on display and packaging tricks to persuade us to buy fabricated food containing waste products and allergenic chemicals. This crisis of human adaptation to the chemical environment, with its terrible implications for health in developed countries, has so far gone almost unnoticed by doctors and politicians. A few of the growing number of people whose health has been affected are showing concern but in most cases even they are too ignorant of the real nature of their predicament to know what to do about it.

We all go into supermarkets or eat convenience foods at some time in our lives; we could all be victims of chemicalized food.

FIVE

My own and other cases

We live in a period of unprecedented environmental change. Breakdown of man's personal powers of adaptation to the ever-increasing load of toxic and allergenic chemicals being put into his food, air and drinking water is already occurring on a massive scale, I believe. People at the more susceptible end of the spectrum of adaptability are now cluttering up hospital beds and doctors' surgeries with illnesses which are neither diagnosed correctly nor treated effectively. Go round the wards of your local mental hospital if you want to see what I mean. Why?

It is not logical immediately to prescribe anti-depressant pills or electro-shock therapy for a girl suffering from suicidal depression without first considering whether her depression might be a manifestation of adaptive breakdown to an environmental hazard like instant coffee or cigarettes, or indeed an undiagnosed attack of tuberculosis or a brain tumour.

Some people seem to think that the instant-prescribing doctor is a new phenomenon. He is not. He has been around since the mid-nineteenth century.

During the year 1877 Dr Robert Bridges, who later, to his patients' relief, gave up medicine to become Poet Laureate, saw 13,940 new patients[26], allotting one minute and sixteen seconds to each. This allowed him time to write various prescriptions suitable to the presenting symptom, e.g. linctus for cough and belladonna for stomach ache. He found this too time-consuming and clipped fourteen seconds off the interview by ordering Blaud's pills for everyone. One variety contained iron, chalk, gum and glucose, another had arsenic added. This gave rise to the complaint, familiar among patients attending NHS doctors today, that 'he doesn't even look up to say hello, he's writing my pre-

cription before I sit down'. Dr Bridges was not exceptional in
those days nor is his kind today, although with the proliferation
of jobs in the NHS the patient may get the impression that he is
being cared for better by social workers, health visitors, district
and community nurses.

No, let's be fair; Robert Bridges was as much a victim of the
system under which he had to practise as is the over-worked
general practitioner or consultant general physician today. Too
many patients chasing doctors with too little time is a sure
prescription for dissatisfaction.

In March 1978 I received a letter from a consultant psychiatrist
on the staff of a neighbouring mental hospital asking if I could
see a girl student, Diana, in his acute admission ward. For two
years Diana's mother, who knew that her daughter was allergic
to eggs and had had allergic exzema badly as a child, had been
asking for someone to explore the possibility that her daughter's
depression might be due to a sort of allergic reaction affecting her
brain.

For medico-political reasons, I could not take Diana back into
Park Prewett, so I offered to drive over to the consultant psychiatrist's hospital and show him and his staff how to test for
food and chemical allergy.

Here is a summary of the case, made soon after she went home
in April 1978:

DIANA K. Twenty-one-year-old female music student, ill
since age thirteen and treated unsuccessfully at various other
hospitals over a period of seven years with psychotropic drugs,
electroshock, group therapy and finally, consignment to a
Richmond Fellowship hostel for mentally disturbed adoles-
cents in Southampton, where she slashed her wrists and was
admitted to hospital.
Main symptoms: depression with weeping, suicide attempts,
tension and inability to sit still, lack of concentration and
drive, loss of libido, poor short-term memory, inability to
read comprehendingly or maintain eye contact. Signs: over-
weight (variable), skin colour changes and oedema of various

parts of body. Cleared on five-day fast with minimal environmental control.

Reacted strongly on challenge with all meats (return of above-
listed symptoms) OK on fresh fruit and vegetables. In hospital
during March 1978. Home since, happy and back in music
studies. Living on unchemically contaminated vegetarian diet.
Non-smoker, non-drinker of alcohol. Not on the contraceptive
pill.

Challenges were done double-blind (see page 58) and with the
following clinical parameters measured: BP, oral temperature,
pulse, respiration, skin colour changes. All or most altered
but main response to active incitant foods was agitation and
loss of eye contact with downcast facial expression.

(*recorded by experienced psychiatric staff nurse*)

In July, Diana sent me a postcard from Switzerland, where she
had gone on holiday with her family, saying how well she
felt. I kept in touch with her and early in 1979 she sent me this
letter:

February 12th, 1979

Dear Dr Mac,

Thank you so much for your Christmas card. We were all
delighted to hear about your research grant – things are looking
up for you too!

You asked how we first discovered it might be chemicals that
I was allergic to, rather than the food itself. I think the idea
came gradually really, probably starting when I tested myself
on milk from goats that were fed organically, soon after coming
home from hospital. Recently we had to change our source of
supply as the lady who had previously sold it to us moved to
Oxford. Again, we made sure that the goat was fed organically,
and again I had no adverse reaction. The woman we now buy
goats' milk from also keeps chickens, organically, and her
husband kills them by strangling, without tranquillizing them.
So, I tried the chicken – no adverse reaction, and the eggs from
the chickens – and again, no adverse reaction. Next, we took up

the offer of a neighbour, whose son-in-law goes shooting, and brings home wild rabbits, hare, pheasant, etc. I have tested all these, with no adverse reaction.

Just recently, we have heard of an organic farm, and we have been given some milk, cream and yogurt, from organically fed cows. We thought this would be the ultimate proof of whether or not it is a chemical allergy – so I tried it. Yet again, there was no adverse reaction. During the last week or so, I have been feeling very slightly tense and on edge, although not depressed in any way. I went on a three-day fast over the weekend and on breaking the fast, the first thing I drank was a large glass of this organic cows' milk, and today I have had chicken and eggs – all from organic sources – and I feel wonderful! Are we right in taking this as positive proof? If so, maybe, one day in the future, it will be possible to find out *which* chemicals affect me, and maybe even find an antidote?

I am still enjoying life to the full. I am sure you will be interested to hear that I have been accepted into the School of Music. I am still taking other auditions in case I decide I'd rather go to a different college, but at least now I know I have *somewhere* to go next September!

I hope things continue to go well for you. I was interested to see you on Southern Television the other day – although I thought they could have given you more time! If there is any way in which I can help you in your research, I would be only too willing.

With very best wishes,

Love,

Diana.

Failure of adaptation to things in the physical environment – foods, drinks and pollutants – is not yet considered by doctors to be a major cause of illness and patients are often too scared or respectful to mention the possibility, when they get to see their doctor.

Dr Théron Randolph of Chicago first put the ecological view

of illness to the British public in 1959 when he was interviewed
by Cliff Michelmore on the BBC programme, 'Tonight'. Here is
a transcript of what he said:

C. M.   Here, to attend the joint CMA meeting in Edinburgh
is Dr Théron G. Randolph. He is participating with Dr
Mitchell of Montreal and a London physician. [*This was me.*]
What is the exhibit?

T. R.   It is a new point of view, that common illnesses are a
result of everyday exposures to which many people are susceptible.

C. M.   What do you mean by 'everyday exposures'?

T. R.   Common foods in the diet – wheat, eggs, milk – never
suspected by the victim – when used everyday in the diet, or
fumes from gas cookers in the kitchen, automobile exhausts
and other chemical odours. Chemical additives and contaminants in food e.g. residue from sprays on the crops.

C. M.   What are the manifestations? How are they ill? What
do they complain of?

T. R.   Fatigue is the cardinal symptom. Then rheumatic pains,
headaches, gastro-intestinal upsets, skin rashes, especially
itching, and most important of all, a large group of mental
symptoms. These include irritability, lack of concentration,
the inability to read comprehendingly. These are at first intermittent and later lead on to continuous depression, confusion
and advanced behaviour disorders which usually lead the
patients into the hands of the psychiatrist.

C. M.   How did you get on the track of all this?

T. R.   This is not original with me. It started with Dr Albert
Rowe in California in the late 20s and 30s. My own interest
developed independently in recording verbatim accounts of my
patients' illnesses on the typewriter. It soon became evident
to me that many common complaints – fatigue, irritability,
muscle and joint pains, occurred in allergy patients who had
come to me for asthma, hay fever and other illnesses ordinarily
recognized as being allergic. As diet was manoeuvred in these
patients for relief of localized allergies, I found that their

general symptoms were relieved also. Moreover, when foods were returned after avoidance, these generalized symptoms were precipitated and appeared in acute recurrences.

C. M. So in fact you were able to use this manipulation of the patients' diet as a means of diagnosis and showing that the cause lay in the taking of common foods?

T. R. Yes, my most effective programme was to isolate a patient in a hospital ward which removed him from home, work and hobbies. He was fasted for four to five days on spring water only, without tobacco or drugs. During this time the symptoms would subside and when the patient was symptom-free, I re-exposed them to the avoided foods one by one, beginning with the common chemically uncontaminated foods. The offending substances were avoided as demonstrated and the patient sent home on a compatible diet on which he could live and feel well. If, on return home, the symptoms came back on this diet, a search was made in the home for possible other substances causing illness.

C. M. Such as?

T. R. Fumes, smells, dust in the home.

C. M. How many people do you think are affected in this way?

T. R. Very many. Perhaps up to eighty per cent of those attending general practitioner surgeries in this country.

C. M. This method of yours seems to involve a complete change in the family doctor's approach to illness.

T. R. Yes, by demonstrating the *cause* of common illnesses, rather than merely treating the symptoms with drugs, my method enables the doctor to help his patient in a more fundamental way. I have found that once this approach is explained to the patients, they are willing and anxious to co-operate in their own rehabilitation.

Randolph is a remarkable man. It is no exaggeration to say that my luck in meeting him changed my life and enabled me to overcome disabilities which could easily have put me out of action. Events which led to my meeting Randolph go back to

1956, a key year for me, because that was when I first suspected food and chemicals of doing something bad to my health.

I developed a temperature with a headache and stiffness at the back of the neck which a GP friend who came to see me diagnosed as meningitis. The neurologist he consulted agreed and wanted to do a lumbar puncture on me. I refused because the extraordinary thing was that I could make the headache go away, temporarily, by drinking strong coffee. After a week or two, the illness subsided.

While I was convalescing, Michael Curtis, the editor of the *News Chronicle*, who, with his family, was on my list of patients, called to see how I was. He found me sitting up in bed feeling better and he said, 'Richard – our doctor on the paper is leaving. Would you like to have a go?' I said I would. That year I was 40 years old. Ever since I had been a boy I had wanted to be a writer. Writing was in the family. The poet Coleridge was a remote ancestor and my grandmother's brother (on my father's side) was Humphrey Milford of the Oxford University Press. But I did not write anything for which I got paid (except advertising copy) until then and after that I followed Dr Samuel Johnson's precept and never wrote anything for which I was *not* paid.

Michael Curtis sent Hugh McLeave, his science correspondent, down to Kew where I had my general practice, to show me how newspaper writing was done and the first piece which appeared over my byline was a feature on the banning of heroin.

By this time, I was feeling more and more depressed and lethargic and getting fatter. I still drank lots of coffee because it seemed to get me going in the morning and pick me up during the day. My weight had gone up to nearly 82 kg (182 lb) which at a height of 167 cm (5′8″) was far too much. I tried cutting down calories, but soon found that boring and ineffective, besides leaving me more tired and depressed. I smoked cigarettes and I drank a fair quantity of alcohol; gin and tonic and wine mainly, with beer and cider for thirst.

To enable me to go regularly to Fleet Street, I managed to persuade a local woman doctor, Betty Macdonald, to assist me part-time in the practice. She was married to James Macdonald,

the ornithologist who was in charge of birds at the Natural
History Museum in South Kensington. The patients all knew her
because she had lived in Kew a long time and she had a fine
combination of canniness with honesty. I felt that I could trust her
absolutely and one of the reasons I gave up the practice eight
years later, in 1964, was that she and James emigrated to Austra-
lia so that he could write a definitive book about Australian
birds. I could not face trying to replace her.

So there I was, with a growing practice, enough money, a
beautiful wife, my son of four years old, and an interesting job
on a national daily, becoming more and more inefficient through
depression and obesity, neither of which I could get the better of.

My job at the *News Chronicle* involved suggesting and writing
features for the middle pages and going in on a Thursday to read
the *Lancet* and *BMJ*, which were sent round by hand from the
printers, for news items which would be in the paper and on their
breakfast tables when doctors received these journals on a Friday.
If the stories were intriguing enough, some doctors actually
opened the journals instead of tossing them, still rolled, into the
pile gathering dust in the corner of the surgery.

On one particular Thursday, in July 1956, as I scanned the
Lancet with lack-lustre eyes, I came on a paper by two re-
searchers, Professor Alan Kekwick and Dr Gaston Pawan at the
Middlesex Hospital Metabolic Unit[21], 'The Effect of Isocaloric
diets on Weight Loss on the Obese'. It really woke me up and I
suggested to the News Editor that I did a piece on it.

'What the hell does it mean?' he asked and I told him that it
meant you could eat as much fat as you liked and still lose
weight, provided you cut down your carbohydrate, *and* you did
not have to count calories. 'Really?' he said. 'That sounds good.
Do me a hundred words.'

My hundred words appeared next day under the headline,
'Cream, Steaks, can make you Slim.'

A three-day feature followed on the eat-fat-grow-slim principle
which involved cutting down carbohydrate to the minimum and
eating fat and protein in the palatable proportion of 1:3. Of
course, I was not the only one to pick up Kekwick and Pawan's

research for my paper. Most of the other nationals did, but none followed it up.

The summary of Kekwick and Pawan's paper was: 'The composition of the diet can alter the expenditure of calories in obese persons, increasing it when fat and proteins are given and decreasing it when carbohydrates are given.'

Meeting Professor Kekwick and Dr Pawan gave me new hope of solving my own obesity problem, and I put myself on a free-calorie high fat, high protein, low carbohydrate diet for three weeks to see what effect it would have. On this diet, which I enjoyed eating and which never left me hungry, I lost 1.35 kg (3 lbs) in three weeks and felt more energetic than I had done for months. Only in the first few days on the diet did I have anything to complain of; a slight headache and some irritability – probably a hangover from all the bread and biscuits which I had been eating before. A book of my findings has been published.[33] (I now know that by cutting out refined carbohydrates I had unintentionally reduced my load of food allergens considerably.)

I embarked for America, to find an American publisher for that book, in November 1958 at Liverpool on the *Empress of England*, which docked at Montreal five days later. One day out from Liverpool I began to feel depressed. It got worse and worse until all I could do was lie on my bunk and read detective stories, between struggling along to meals which seemed to pick me up for an hour or two, then the gloom descended again. It was not a rough crossing and in any case I never suffer from motion sickness. Nor was it the food, because with the wide choice offered by Canadian Pacific, it was easy to follow the same diet I had been on at home.

There was a good crowd of people on board but I could not face any of them. Looking back, I think this was an acute manifastation of my allergy to petrochemicals. The *Empress* had been newly painted and the smell of paint, plus the usual shipboard fumes of oil, tar and synthetic fabrics affected my brain. Solvents used in paint are among the most allergenic of all the chemicals affecting the central nervous system. One of my patients goes into an epilepsy-like seizure on entering a newly painted room; another becomes acutely depressed and suicidal. These solvents are fractions of the distillate from crude oil; the best known is white spirit which comes off at 60°C (140°F). Paints giving harder or fancier finishes contain stronger solvents like toluene and xylene (both poisonous) and some contain oils modified with isocyanate, a cyanide compound of great toxicity which should never be applied in an unventilated room.

I noticed also a phenomenon, which I now know to be allergic, in one of the pursers at whose table I sat for meals. He used to come to breakfast silent and glum until they brought his usual two boiled eggs. Soon after eating these he perked up, became chatty and was able to smile. The overnight avoidance of egg had got him into the hangover zone from them and he had to wait for more before he could get back to normal.

In Montreal, I stayed with Ray Lawson, surgeon to the Canadian Arctic Medical Service (the flying doctor service for the far north) and an authority on the Eskimo and his high fat, non-carbohydrate way of eating. At a party he gave for me to meet some of his colleagues, one in particular wanted to talk to me. He was Dr Donald Mitchell, a dermatologist and brother-in-law to Dr Théron Randolph, the Chicago allergist. He told me that he had read my book[33] and wondered why I had not mentioned food allergy as a major cause of obesity through addictive eating of allergenic, carbohydrate foods. I told him I had never heard of food allergy, so he filled me in a little and persuaded me to change my route so as to take in a visit to Ted Randolph in Chicago, on my way to New York.

The Randolphs' flat in Chicago was unusual; no carpets, just unpolished, stripped-wood floors. All upholstery and hangings in cloth made from fibres of natural origin; wool or cotton. All windows shut and fitted with electrostatic, carbon filters, so that the air felt clean after the stinky Chicago streets. The heating and cooking was all electric; no gas in the building at all, because gas utilities are high on the list of offenders with chemical-allergic people.

The flat was on the twentieth floor of a block of apartments (they now live on the fiftieth, in a block on a bit of land jutting out into the lake and buffetted by high winds – about the least polluted position in Chicago). It was my first encounter with an ecological living place designed to minimize atmospheric pollution; the kind of chemical-free oasis all chemical victims have to aim to live in if they are to remain well in our increasingly polluted cities.

The Randolphs are chemical victims themselves, she more than he. Driving with them into Chicago on my last visit in 1977 from Zion where Ted has his Ecology Unit in the International Hospital, Ted drove with a portable air filter between the front seats and all the windows closed. The car was an old Mercedes with leather upholstery and a stainless steel, non-corrodable exhaust system. In 1958, on this first visit, good portable air filters for car interiors had not been developed and Mrs Randolph had to use a respirator in the worst of the downtown traffic.

At that time Ted Randolph was not the widely-known, respected figure that he is now. He worked at the Swedish Covenant Hospital in a not very smart part of Chicago and he was encountering the kind of opposition from his medical colleagues that I have, until very recently.

He had not more than half-a-dozen rooms allotted to him in which to treat patients, and no office for himself, so that he had to interview patients and their relatives on a corridor. Nevertheless, his nurses were loyal and he was getting some spectacular results with all sorts of chronic ailments – rheumatism, migraine, colitis, depression for example – using an initial fast on nothing but spring water and then, if the symptoms cleared, challenging the patients first with organic and then with commercial versions of the foods they had been eating served one at a time as single portions, four or five hours apart.

This two-stage testing distinguished between allergy to foods per se and allergy to the chemicals put into them by the grower or manufacturer. Foods had to be chosen which were readily available in both forms, e.g. peaches, cherries, salmon, broccoli, apple, celery and lettuce, which during its growing period is sprayed up to fourteen times with pesticides.

He told me that extremely chemical-susceptible patients showed acute reactions after the first feeding with a chemically contaminated food, but that less susceptible people needed two or three days of cumulative ingestion before they showed convincing reactions. He emphasized that allergy to plain or source foods and to their chemical contaminants can give rise to identical symptoms, though those associated with chemicals tended to be more severe.

Randolph showed me many cases. Some were of food allergy only, and fairly simple to work out; others were mainly chemical and I will describe one in detail because it was the first one I had seen demonstrated and was so dramatic that it started me looking for evidence of chemical allergy in my own case and in a number of puzzling patients in my practice in Kew. This case is described at length in Randolph's book.[44] I was able to see and talk to the patient and I saw her become unconscious when she was accidentally exposed to a few puffs of a perfumed aerosol.

Mrs K. P., aged forty-four, housewife, was first seen by Randolph in 1953. As a child she was hyperactive and jittery, with bouts of runny nose, sick headache and car sickness. These symptoms were usually treated with aspirin and later with antihistamines. All her symptoms were worse in the kitchen where she became clumsy and broke dishes, crying when reproached. She preferred to stay out of doors, where she said there was more air.

Throughout her childhood, she was never able to concentrate for long on anything at home, while at school her work was erratic, with some good days and some bad, on which she could not recall what she had previously learnt. In retrospect it seems that she was always worse in rooms heated with unvented kerosene (paraffin) stoves, lit by kerosene lamps, and in kitchens with gas or kerosene cookers.

On moving from the country into Chicago at the age of fifteen, all her symptoms became worse, and worse still, on moving into a newly-painted flat in 1944. Intermittent colds and influenza occurred throughout that winter. Food allergy was suspected after each attempt to eat cherries, although she has since eaten organically grown, chemically uncontaminated cherries without trouble.

The following summer in camp, even though eating all foods available, she remained well until she was given sulphonamides as a protection against scarlet fever with which she had come into contact. Immediately following this she developed nausea and extreme listlessness.

With the onset of the cool weather in the autumn, she spent more time indoors and suffered a recurrence of runny nose, bronchitis and fevers, for which she was given sulphonamides a second time.* This was followed by a rash all over her body so the drug had to be stopped. Later that autumn, she enrolled in a pottery class but found that her respiratory symptoms increased and she developed asthma, whenever they opened the gas-fired kiln. So she had to drop out of pottery class, although she liked it.

All through that winter she continued to have asthma intermittently, unexplained fevers and extreme fatigue which only made her feel worse. During the winter of 1945/46, she was diagnosed as having influenza seven times. She had constant headaches and because of loss of appetite, nausea and vomiting, she lost 11.25 kg (25 lbs) in one month. During this time she was on daily doses of pain-killers and barbiturates (sedatives) and this continued for seven years.

Coincident with this day-in, day-out medication, her symptoms changed from seasonal to perennial and although she was suspected of being sensitive to certain drugs, there was little change in her condition when some of these were discontinued singly. By this time she was aware of acute sensitivity to procain (local anaesthetic), synthetic vitamin B and several antibiotics.

On moving into an old house in the autumn of 1947 and painting the interior herself, her asthma and bronchitis became much worse. In the spring of 1948, a major gas leak was detected in her stove and she found she could get temporary relief from her respiratory symptoms by deliberately inhaling the heated air from

*It is not uncommon for the same chemical to produce different symptoms on different occasions in the same patient.

her gas oven; she inhaled this repeatedly whenever she had an asthmatic attack.

Although she could get temporary relief of asthma from her gas cooker, she got more headaches, staggering, intermittent losses of consciousness and pains in her muscles and joints. So the 'hair of the dog' treatment with gas was not exactly a cure-all.

In the summers when she could be out of doors she improved and in the winters she got worse until, after the usual spell of invalidism in the winter of 1949/50, she was taken to a ranch in Arizona, where within a week she got better. Short episodes of asthma, headache and rheumatic pain occurred on very cold days when she had to stay indoors with the unvented, gas wall heater on.

She became ill when she went home and remained so except for the odd occasion when she went camping or could stay out side most of the time.

Remember that in the early 1950s chemical air pollution was not suspected. As her illness progressed, Mrs K. P. became more and more disabled, with episodes of hyperactivity, inability to speak and confusion suggesting alcoholic intoxication (in fact she was tee-total). She was frequently hospitalized in semi-conscious, depressed stupor and became almost symptom-free by the third or fourth day if the hospital had no gas. It was costing her and her family a small fortune. Eventually, when she was about to be committed compulsorily to a mental institution, someone sent her to Dr Randolph, who soon recognized the probable chemical origin of her symptoms.

A neurologist saw her at the beginning of her stuporose phase and strongly suspected hysteria. When I saw her she was having her food and chemical sensitivites (allergies) worked out by Dr Randolph. Here was a patient who would undoubtedly have spent the rest of her life as a compulsory patient in a mental hospital. Mrs K. P. was the first case of severe allergy to domestic gas and other inhalant chemicals which Randolph showed me. When I went back in 1963, I saw many more chemical victims.

Let me explain this addictive, 'hair of the dog' phenomenon in allergy both to foods and chemicals, which was introduced briefly in this case.

The fact that susceptible people are first picked-up or stimulated and later hung-over (made ill) by frequent exposure to the thing to which they have developed allergy has lately been grasped and written about by popular journalists. I first explained it for the non-medical reader in 1959 in an article in the *News Chronicle* and later in *Today* magazine (a dolled-up version of the old *John Bull*) in 1961, under the headline 'Hangovers from Food'.

Understanding of this masking by temporary allergic stimulation (see page 24) answers the commonest question I am asked about food allergy: 'How can people possibly be allergic to common foods which they eat and enjoy every day?'

Writing in the March 1979 number of *Woman's Journal*, Celia Hall described masking. A chronic, fluctuating level of symptoms will persist when a person is partially adapting to an allergic food eaten day after day. He will feel relatively well immediately after a meal containing that food and will develop symptoms some hours later, unless the food has been eaten again. This is called masking.

Total avoidance of the food for more than three days will render him hypersensitive so that another dose of it, either accidentally or by deliberate challenge, will produce an obvious reaction. A further smaller dose of the same food will turn the reaction off, i.e. will mask the symptoms again.

Susan Todd, a staff nurse on one of the acute admission wards at my hospital, used her knowledge of masking to avert a catastrophe which might have led to a patient's suicide. I will call the patient Pauline.

A fire had broken out on the ward and the patients had to be evacuated in a hurry. When the fire was put out and the patients had come back, the first thing they all wanted after the excitement and panic was a cup of tea. So some of them went into the kitchen and brewed up. Before the nurses or anyone else in the know could intervene Pauline had been handed a mug of hot, sweet tea and began to drink it. (Sugar was one of her troublemakers, which she had avoided for several weeks.) The reaction was almost instantaneous. She began to cry and then had to be held down in her chair by three nurses to prevent her from trying to injure herself which she had so often done.

Sue Todd realized what had happened and quickly mixed some sugar and water in a spoon. She forced it between Pauline's lips. Within a minute she had calmed down and soon was looking round, smiling at everyone and asking what all the fuss was about. If she had been unsupervised she might have tried to injure herself. The 'turn-off' dose in such a situation needs to be quite small; in fact if it can be gauged very precisely, that dose can be used prophylactically (as a protection) dropped under the tongue twice or three times a week, or injected into the skin as a form of desensitization, thus enabling a patient to eat a food to which they have become allergic, without getting sick.

The same thing can be done with chemicals, and later, when I deal with prevention and treatment of allergy for the chemical victim, these methods will be described in detail. It is possible now, using the right apparatus and technique, to protect oneself against allergy to any food or chemical, from bread and strawberries to North Sea gas and synthetic dress materials. Recently I have been given a research grant to buy equipment for making extracts of various allergenic foods and chemical-derived household materials with which to diagnose patients' allergies and make up de-sensitizing injections and sub-lingual drops with which to keep them well.

The apparatus consists of millipore filters for preparing sterile extracts of things like plastic floor tiles, household dust and cleaning materials, with syringes, needles and hundreds of rubber-capped bottles in which to make serial dilutions of the extracts.

Doctors in America have been working along these lines since the 1950s. In 1964, Dr Marshall Mandell of Norwalk, Connecticut, told me of his first experience with the method. A little girl was brought to his office in an acute asthmatic attack, blue in the face and fighting for breath. She had been standing by her father while he painted a wooden fence with creosote, when she started to wheeze. As she was a known allergic asthmatic, they rushed her off to Dr Mandell. He tried to turn her asthma off with creosote, diluting some with water, then putting one drop under the girl's tongue. Much to his relief, her asthmatic attack ended abruptly and she was able to go home. Creosote contains phenol (carbolic), a basic petrochemical to which many people are allergic and which can be used in minute quantities to desensitize chemically allergic people.

As the masking and unmasking of food and chemical allergy is such an important phenomenon to understand, I am going to quote a piece about it from an article which I wrote with Sue Todd.[53] It tells how the masking of responses to an allergen, or any potentially harmful substance, can be explained in terms of stress (the battle to remain normal in the face of any noxious agent). Adaptation is the key to food and chemical allergy. Since the early 1930s, Hans Selye, Professor of Experimental Medicine and Surgery at the University of Montreal, has studied the mechanisms underlying the adaptation of living creatures to harmful agents. He has become the world's leading authority on stress and the diseases of adaptation.

In 1936 he published a brief account of his work on experimental animals, using stress-inducing agents of several kinds; including heat, cold and toxic substances. Later, he added allergens to the stressors studies (Selye, 1946).[51]

He found that all living organisms responded in a general, three-stage way; first showing *alarm* and going into what might be likened to surgical shock; second, recovering and moving into a stage of resistance (or adaptation) after a few days, if the stressing agent continued to be applied.

Third, (much later) they passed into an exhaustion stage from which recovery did not occur because adaptive resources based on pituitary and adrenal hormones were worn out.

In 1956, Professor Adolph[1] in New York, reported stages of adaptation similar to those described by Selye but found that individual animals showed marked differences in their responses to the same stressful agent.

Thus was born the specific adaptation syndrome, a phrase

coined by Randolph to explain Rinkel's masking phenomenon (see page 24).

Taking the stressor substance to be a common food or chemical to which allergy has developed, each widely spaced exposure to that substance will be followed by an immediate onset of symptoms. This is the stage of alarm (stage 1).

Now if the rate or exposure or ingestion is increased to daily or more often, adaptive responses will come into play which ensure that the subject feels good or even better than usual, after each exposure (stage 2A).

This is masking as defined by Rinkel above, and is the basis of food addiction.

Suppose the allergenic food is cow's milk. At first, the baby will vomit or show abdominal distress immediately on ingestion, but if the mother persists with cow's milk feeding, a reversal of these effects will occur.

Now, only if she *stops* giving cow's milk to the baby for a day will it become upset with withdrawal symptoms, which can be relieved by feeding with milk within three days (this is the 'hair of the dog' phenomenon seen in all types of addiction, including food addiction).

Eventually, after some years, a transition stage will be entered (stage 2B) in which more and more of the addictant or allergenic food is needed to maintain the picked-up state, and symptoms will come on more frequently, unless resort is made more and more often to larger and larger doses of the food responsible.

Finally, stage 3, the stage of exhaustion will be reached, when the child will react adversely, immediately (as in stage 1) to every feeding of cow's milk. Stage 3 is more often approached than entered, because symptoms occur fairly often in the transition period of stage 2. Medical help is sought because of the intermittent bouts of illness.

Identification of a causative, common food allergen is made by five days avoidance of the suspect food (during which all withdrawal symptoms clear), followed by test re-exposure by sub-lingual or intradermal challenge, which will produce an

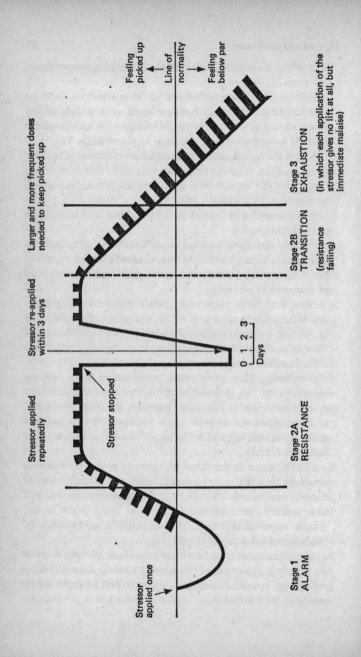

Feeling picked up ← Line of normality → Feeling below par

Stressor applied once

Stage 1 ALARM

Stressor applied repeatedly

Stressor stopped

Stage 2A RESISTANCE

Days 0 1 2 3

Stressor re-applied within 3 days

Stage 2B TRANSITION (resistance failing)

Larger and more frequent doses needed to keep picked up

Stage 3 EXHAUSTION (in which each application of the stressor gives no lift at all, but immediate malaise) immediate, acute and convincing reaction within a few minutes. If the test food is eaten and swallowed in the normal way, a reaction may not be seen for 20 to 30 minutes.

During the five-day fast, the patient will have been taken from the end of stage 2, or the beginning of stage 3, back to stage 1, in which challenge will cause disturbance in one or more systems of the body; a demonstrable, repeatable diagnostic procedure.

The realization that gas was a major factor in my illness came slowly. Randolph had told me of the possibility, and my wife had often remarked how tired *she* felt after spending time in the room where she dried the baby's clothes on an unvented gas heater. In the winter, when I spent long hours in my study and surgery with gas fires burning, I used to become so lethargic and depressed that I could scarcely think straight. Working out in the garden in spring seemed to put me temporarily right.

The key to my own health problem (obesity and depression) was food and chemical allergy and after meeting Randolph I set about putting into practice what he had taught me in order to get my weight down permanently and defeat the depression which had haunted me since I was twenty. To do this I began to re-structure my diet and my house, with particular emphasis on the removal of all gas and oil-burning appliances. Ironically, just before I went over to America we had had new gas fires and a cooker put in! We found an all-electric house on Kew Green but I had to continue the practice at the old house in Kew Road where the ancient gas meter was in the basement, right under the floor of my surgery. I kidded myself that I could get away with it, and with drinking quite large amounts of beer and gin. But I was wrong.

In the winter of 1962 I was hit by the worst depression I had ever had and determined to go back to Chicago and stay with Randolph to get my food allergies worked out. He kindly agreed

Fig. 1. The stages of adaptation involved when an allergy develops to a stressor substance, such as a common food or chemical. (By courtesy of *Nursing Times*).

to have me, put me in the attic of his house out of everybody's
way, with a desk and a truckle bed. There I did a ten-day fast
on nothing but bottled spring water to drink. I kept a diary and
by the third day my black mood had lifted and I began to feel
life was worth living again.

Challenges with the foods I had been eating regularly in the
past revealed several sensitivities: to eggs, coffee and cereal grains
especially. With the exclusion of these and with no gas (the
Randolph's house had none) I became incredibly well. I lost over
a stone in weight and my energy and mental acuity was better
than I could ever remember.

I went off on a tour with Ted Randolph to meet among others
Rachel Carson, author of *Silent Spring*.[7] I remember her as a
frail, pale, gentle person, sitting in the drawing room looking
out on her beautiful Maryland garden, taking China tea with us
and talking about the connections between her book and Ted's[44]
which had been published that year.

In all her work, her main interest had been the relation of life
to its environment and since 1958 she had been collecting data
from doctors and scientists all over the world about the dangers
of synthetic insecticides like DDT and Malathion which are
poisonous to the human liver and central nervous system. Her
medical knowledge was wide and I discovered on reading her
book later that she was well aware of the danger of allergy to
chemicals:

Why does not everyone handling and using insecticides develop
the same symptoms? Here the matter of individual sensitivity
enters in. There is some evidence that women are more susceptible than men, the very young more than adults, those who
lead sedentary, indoor lives more than those leading a rugged
life of work or exercise in the open. Beyond these differences
are others that are no less real because they are intangible.
What makes one person allergic to dust or pollen, sensitive
to a poison, or susceptible to an infection whereas another is
not is a medical mystery for which there is at present no explanation. The problem nevertheless exists and it affects

significant numbers of the population. Some physicians estimate that a third or more of their patients show signs of some form of sensitivity, and that the number is growing. And, unfortunately, sensitivity may suddenly develop in a person previously insensitive. In fact, some medical men believe that intermittent exposures to chemicals may produce just such sensitivity. If this is true, it may explain why some studies on men subjected to continuous occupational exposure find little evidence of toxic effects. By their constant contact with the chemicals these men keep themselves desensitized by repeated small injections of the allergen.

The whole problem of pesticide poisoning is enormously complicated by the fact that a human being, unlike a laboratory animal living under rigidly controlled conditions, is never exposed to one chemical alone. Between the major groups of insecticides, and between them and other chemicals, there are interactions that have serious potentials. Whether released into soil or water or a man's blood, these unrelated chemicals do not remain segregated; there are mysterious and unseen changes by which one alters the power of another for harm.

SIX

Drugs as toxins

Chemical pollution of the individual is not just an accidental by-product of the industrialization of food. Society and the environment have become industrialized also. Some of this pollution is being actively prescribed and this worries many thoughtful doctors who see the results in mental disturbance, drug addiction and the heavy loss of life and limb on the roads.

For practical purposes, all drugs are toxic in overdose, but overdose is relative. A dose which is harmless to one person may be almost lethal to another because of allergy, kidney disease (imparing excretion) or liver damage (imparing detoxification).

One woman in every five in Britain takes a tranquillizer at some time during each year. Dr John Clarke, until recently, honorary secretary of the Police Surgeons' Association, said: 'Surveys have shown that fifteen per cent of drivers on the road are under the influence of drugs at any given time. Night time sedation and tranquillizers are turning drivers into potential killers.'

The word 'tranquillizer' was invented by the pharmaceutical industry to describe a new class of drug, introduced to doctors in the early 1950s, which was claimed to calm down anxious patients without making them drowsy.

Before the invention of tranquillizers like Valium, Librium, and the rest, small doses of sedatives, sleeping pills or hypnotics such as Medinal and Amytal (barbiturates) were prescribed for anxious patients to take during the daytime.

With the coming of the tranquillizers many of the dangers associated with daytime sedation with hypnotic drugs were reduced; e.g. impaired concentration, falling asleep at the wheel of a car, or general lack of alertness.

There is no doubt that tranquillizers are less dangerous than sedatives for daytime use, but it is wrong to claim that they do not cloud consciousness at all. Many people are made slightly dopey by them, and some blunting of appropriate emotional responses occurs, which can impoverish relationships with others and reduce overall mental acuity. And, like all drugs which act on the brain, they can be addictive.

Not only sedatives and tranquillizers but all drugs with an action on the central nervous system can cause accidents, and that includes the widely prescribed antihistamines given for allergy and travel sickness.

In 1975, the last year for which figures are available, more than fifty million prescriptions were issued in England and Wales for sleeping pills, tranquillizers, anti-depressants, antihistamines and stimulants.

Dr Andrew Raffle, Chairman of the Medical Commission on Accident Prevention, addressing a Pharmaceutical Society symposium on drugs and driving in 1977, told of a doctor who had taken a carefully prescribed dose of antihistamine for his hay fever. Later he found himself driving straight for a traffic island, laughing his head off.

Dr William Reilly, a Shropshire GP, in an article in the *British Medical Journal* in 1975 on drugs and driving, gave the following story, and several more: A woman discharged from a mental hospital, having been prescribed five different pills affecting her central nervous system, drove to his surgery and arrived in an obviously drugged state. Despite his warnings, she insisted on driving home.

Just how profoundly drugs prescribed for all sorts of conditions can affect consciousness and powers of judgement, is not fully appreciated, even by doctors.

Recently, when I was Duty Psychiatrist at the hospital I was called to the Surgical Floor in the general division to see an old lady of seventy-four, who had come through a gall-bladder operation successfully and had then been noticed by the nurses to have gone mad. There was no doubt that she was deluded and having visual hallucinations. Her husband, who was a good deal older, but still apparently well, was sitting beside the bed and I asked him to stay and interpret for me because it was difficult to make head or tail of the rubbish she was talking.

He told me that before she came in for her operation she had been 'seeing things' that were not there; rats and rabbits in the bedroom at night and that sort of thing. No amount of reasoning by him had had any effect in shaking her conviction that these hallucinations were real.

Well, I knew from many years in psychiatry and before that as a GP, that visual hallucinations are nearly always a sign of organic brain disturbance, most commonly nowadays from drugs.

I was surprised to see the number of drugs for which she was written up. The new and junior house surgeon had just copied off the long list that her GP had sent in with her. It included a notorious precipitator of delusions and hallucinations called levodopa or L-dopa (hailed on its first introduction as the wonder drug for Parkinsonism or paralysis agitans).

There was no evidence that she had had Parkinson's disease so perhaps the GP had added it to her list because she had arterio-sclerosis which can cause Parkinsonism. I stopped the L-dopa along with several other drugs which seemed to me to be unnecessary, and within a day or two her mind cleared and she became a charming old lady, somewhat puzzled and faintly self-deprecating about the rats and rabbits which she now realized had probably not been jumping on to her bed. Follow-up at home after she went out was arranged with the Community Nursing Service and so far she has remained well, since she has ceased to take the drugs which were affecting her brain, either through allergy or poisoning.

On 5 October 1978, Westminster Hospital Medical School in London put on a symposium on iatrogenic disease as part of the annual Old Students' Day. The Professor of Medicine, Malcolm Milne, who chaired the meeting, defined iatrogenic disease as that caused by doctors, and told a story about a certain Lieutenant George Simmons wounded at the battle of Waterloo, 15 June 1815. He was hit in the back by a French sniper. The ball lodged near his right nipple and was removed by an army surgeon who bled him of a quart of blood. He was evacuated to Brussels, fifteen miles away, and just survived the journey on horseback. Comfortably billeted with friends and attended by his batman he might have made an uneventful recovery. But the army doctors insisted on bleeding him several times, which made him so ill that his servant took to secretly burying the leeches he was supposed to supply in the garden. Simmons by this time was in and out of stupor, pale and near death. At last, on 14 July, his wound burst, discharging a large quantity of pus. He survived to the time of the Crimean war, but, fortunately, was too old to serve. Diagnosis: exsanguination shock. He was a victim of the treatments fashionable at the time. Today he might have been a chemical victim.

Subsequent speakers at the Westminster symposium gave modern examples of iatrogenesis. Skin specialist Dr Peter Samman dealt with misuse of topical steroids (locally applied ointments containing cortisone-like compounds). These are now the most widely prescribed class of drugs in dermatology. When used for the treatment of peri-oral or rosaceous dermatitis (an allergic condition), steroid ointments control the rash for a while; suddenly some patients can develop a persistent pustular eruption – the steroid face. Tetracycline, an antibiotic also liable to cause allergy, is the recommended antidote.

Ointments are more readily absorbed through the skin than creams or lotions and 25 grammes of a well-known proprietary steroid ointment per week (quite a small tube) will be enough to cause weight gain, striae (stretch marks), raised blood pressure, water retention, dowager's hump, moon face and gross aggravation of any infection. 'Impetigo goes wild,' said Dr Samman.

Doctors have become so accustomed to prescribing potent drugs for any and every condition that they tend to overlook the potential and serious side effects which the drugs may have. Apart from all those just listed, the marked heightening of sexual appetite which steroids often cause can be awkward, as you can imagine. Taken for long periods by mouth, steroids can even cause insanity and death.

In 1961, in an article which I wrote for *Today* magazine, I

predicted trouble for President Kennedy from the steroids he had
been taking ever since he suffered adrenal failure as a result of
swimming while towing an injured crewman several miles in the
China seas after their ship was sunk.

Some of the side effects mentioned were already beginning to
show by the time he was shot dead in Dallas. So it is possible
that drug idiosyncrasies could alter the course of history.

Dr Peter Dally, consultant psychiatrist at Westminster, gave a
talk on psychotropic drugs (anti-depressants and tranquillizers).
He said that seventy-five per cent of suicide *attempts* are now
made with these drugs, 1,600 coming into his hospital per year
for resuscitation and 800 being seen as out-patients. These figures
are by no means exceptional. Multiply them by the number of
equivalent-sized hospitals in the country and you have a sizeable
problem with iatrogenic attempted suicide. Tranquillizers and
anti-depressants were introduced in the mid-1950s. Since then,
their popularity has increased year by year. They are prescribed,
and indeed demanded by patients, because there is now a widespread conviction that extremes of feeling, engendered by the
ordinary stresses of life, are best dealt with by medication. This
damping down or 'normalizing' of emotional responses by mood-
altering drugs is often bad medicine. There are times when they
may be needed for short periods but there is rarely any justification for continuing them for months. When an allergic reaction
affecting the brain can be demonstrated, the treatment should
be tailored to this diagnosis.

All drugs are designed to alter the biochemistry of the body;
many are lethal if taken in overdose and a bottle of fifty amitryp-
tilline tablets (an anti-depressant popular with GPs and psychiatrists) if taken all at once, will put you in a coma from which the
casualty department of your local hospital will have a hard job
resuscitating you. It is not generally known that this class of drug
is chemically related to the antihistamines, developed to combat
allergy.

Could it be that the undoubted success that these drugs have
in relieving anxiety and depression is in some way related to their
anti-allergic properties? This could be a clue to the allergic or

ecological nature of much mental disturbance.

Both allergy and the side effects of drugs can be explained in terms of biochemical variations between one person and another. Hippocrates spoke of 'that infinitely variable organism without which human disease is impossible'. Just as it takes two to make a case of infectious illness (the victim and the bug), so it takes two to respond well or adversely to the prescribed remedy, the patient and the drug.

The whole subject of biochemical individuality is dealt with admirably by Dr Roger J. Williams, co-founder of the Clayton Foundation Biochemical Institute at the University of Texas, in his book.[56] His interest in human biochemical variability was aroused 20 years earlier by the observation that creatine, a chemical substance which tastes bitter to some, is absolutely tasteless to others. He also noticed that some apparently normal individuals were unable to detect the odour of skunk. I have drawn heavily on the ideas in this book for what I am saying in the next few pages.

Krantz and Carr in their book on pharmacology and medical practice[24] admit frankly that 'the mechanism of idiosyncracy is not understood'. The chemistry of a drug or food additive may be known but the chemistry of the living organism with which it interacts is much more obscure, so that idiosyncracy can be neither anticipated nor fully explained.

It has been stated that almost three per cent of all admissions to hospital are due to adverse drug reactions and another two per cent to overdosage.[17] This may understate the problem because it does not include the proportion of patients, like the one I quoted earlier, who get better simply by having drugs stopped when they come into hospital, or the ten to fifteen per cent who develop adverse reactions to drugs during their stay on the wards. The search for a completely safe drug is a pipe dream, satirized by Aldous Huxley in *Brave New World*[19] in which a totally harmless tranquillizer, 'soma', was fed to the toiling masses; and also satirized in this parody of a well-known Anglican hymn:

'Build me newer molecules
Oh my soul –
As the swift seasons roll
Let each new compound
Safer than the last
Avoid reactions observed in the past
Till all at length are free
From vexing idiosyncrasy.'
(*attributed by Roger Williams to Dragstedt*)

This discussion of prescribed drugs and their idiosyncratic side effects is intended to point out the danger of causing damage and creating allergy in people susceptible to chemicals, *not* to condemn the pharmaceutical industry for its enterprise which has provided us with specific remedies for many lethal infections and above all for acute pain, both mental and physical.

Acceptance of the single-cause single-effect approach to medicine and science is one of the presuppositions of technological society. Without it, doctors and scientists would have difficulty communicating with the public, who fund their research and still accept this simplistic view of illness and treatment, because journalists report medical and scientific work in these terms. Here in 1972 *Reader's Digest* said[46]:

The Inter-Society Commission for Heart Disease Resources recommended a five to ten year controlled study, involving 100,000 persons, to determine once and for all whether cutting out fats can reduce the horrendous heart disease toll.

How on earth do you persuade 100,000 people not to eat fat for 10 years? The tragedy is, that just when chemical contamination of our food, water and indoor air is making more and more people vaguely ill with all-over symptoms, doctors are becoming less inclined to look for causes in the environment and more resourceful in fractionating the patient down to his constituent parts looking for 'real' (often irreversible) changes which match the pathology taught in medical school and can be attributed to single causes.

The old-style family physician used to go into the patient's home and make recommendations about diet, heating, ventilation and physical surroundings. Since the Second World War, as the general practitioner has withdrawn into his practice premises, and cut down on house calls, the patient has been left to cope without medical guidance with an increasingly dangerous personal environment.

The following case history illustrates the need for surveillance of the chemical environment and exclusion of specific food allergens, in preference to magic-bullet prescribing and last-resort surgery.

'I became ill in 1971. Ulcerative colitis and Crohn's disease. The diagnosis was slow, X-rays proved inconclusive. Blood loss was heavy and I remember I lay in bed and watched the snow of winter turn to spring. By the summer, I seriously wondered whether I would see Christmas. Hospital treatment and drugs proved only marginally effective, except for large doses of steroids, which brought many undersirable side effects.

I was sent home with a diet sheet (at least the hospital has now torn this up!). I had always wondered about the food I was eating. I spent weeks, months, even a couple of years trying to discover some food that was upsetting me. If I ate nothing for a day or two, I felt drastically worse. (I now know this to be a "hangover symptom" from a masked allergy.) Gradually, as the disease progressed, a sort of depression set in. I became confused, apathetic and developed a strange sort of writer's cramp – I just couldn't write. It was at this time that I heard of Dr Mackarness, his book and his work. He has shown how allergies can be hidden and most important of all, how to unmask them. At first it seemed incredible that such things as milk and white flour can make one so ill, physically and mentally. Doctors have treated allergies for pollen, dust, even trees. Dr Mac has shown how food and its chemical additives can cause much misery. I am now better but there is much to be done. We must make food testing quicker, easier and far more accessible, and we must find ways of tackling the chemical problem.'

This man, who we will call David, is a graphic designer and a member of the Chemical Victims Club. He wrote this optimistic instalment of his history not long after I had worked out his food sensitivities at a time when he was feeling pretty well. Before that, he had managed to persuade the junior doctor who was seeing him to reduce his steroid drugs and try the allergy-blocking agent, Nalcrom.* This young doctor's chief was against stopping steroids and was arranging for David's colon to be removed by a surgical colleague. But, because of the depression which had come to figure in David's clinical picture, a psychiatric opinion had been sought, and as Duty Psychiatrist the day this happened, the case was referred to me.

After seeing David, I decided to try to get him under my care, in order to study his food allergies and get him off steroids. The physician and the surgeon who had been looking after him were happy for me to do this and stipulated only that I should send him back to them if I failed and the colectomy operation became necessary.

So he came into a side room on the medical floor at Basingstoke in 1976 and I was able to show that his colon reacted with pain, bleeding and diarrhoea on challenge with heavily chemicalized foods like white flour and battery farm chicken. Untreated foods like lamb and organically grown fruit and vegetables caused no trouble.

He was well when he went home but developed headache, depression and fatigue on returning to the studio where he worked. I kept in touch with him and he sent me this letter:

Wed Aug 23rd 1978

As promised, a short account of how the world is treating me, at the moment. After being 'worked out' at Basingstoke Hospital, I've a pretty good idea of all the foods that upset me. At least people who are allergic to foods can avoid them; not so the ever-increasing barrage of air pollutants. Sprays,

---

*Fison's trademark name for orally active sodium chromoglycate, already well-known as Intal, the form in which it is prescribed to prevent allergic asthma (see pages 57–63).

smoke, engine fumes, polishes, all conspire to make life a
misery for more people than can ever be appreciated by a
gullible (progress-seeking?) public. As you know, at my place
of employment, we suffer the fumes of printing inks and white
spirit, turps. etc. You will appreciate that having worked out
a suitable diet, it is much easier to tell just what if anything
makes me feel unwell. I felt really well for the three weeks I
was away from the firm on annual holiday. On returning, for
the first hour or so – ok but by mid-morning I felt sick and
faint with quite a headache.

Gradually, of course this goes and one only feels ill in the
early evening, after leaving work; the whole cycle to be repeated the next day. At this point I realize the sceptic might
well diagnose an allergy to *work* rather than its environment.

This week the boss and a lot of our artists are on holiday,
so I have had the lads in our studio seal up all the containers,
inks and paints etc. and store them all away. (I should point
out it is not necessary to use them all the time, and I never use
them personally.) Guess what? No symptoms but still plenty
of work!

It occurs to me that many of our lads have been made ill
by this stuff, one having part of his colon removed, but usually
we all just get addicted to it and many can plod on for years
before becoming seriously ill.

Well, that's about it. I hope you are well, I know you are
busy. See you soon.

Yours chemically smitten,
David.

David's case illustrates the two main routes by which environmental chemicals can impinge on the health of the individual,
breaking down his powers of adaptation; via his food or the air
he breathes. In hospital he was given challenge feedings with
various foods. Battery raised chicken caused David's colon to
go into spasm and bleed, and his own experiment at work proved
that air-borne fumes of inks, paint and turpentine were causing
his faintness and sick headaches.

Both David, upset by supermarket chicken, and Diana (see page 69) made ill by mass-produced eggs, lead us to look at commercial chicken farming. Margaret Lane, asking 'Did you enjoy your breakfast?' in an article in the *Sunday Telegraph*,[28] on where eggs and hens come from, wrote:

> There were three battery houses each containing 2,800 birds. In each aisle there were three layers of wire cages; the top layer had the benefit of cobweb-festooned electric light, the middle layer was dim and the bottom layer in virtual darkness. The cages measured 46 cm (18 in) by 41 cm (16 in) each containing six birds, so closely packed that it was almost impossible to move, let alone flap or stretch a wing. The stench and the noise, the thousands of clacking heads straining out through the wire, made the place seem like hell.
>
> All the birds' necks were naked of feathers, since they must thrust their heads through the wire to reach food or obtain a drop of water from an overhead nozzle ... during the twelve months they inhabit their cells and despite suffocating stench and din, the birds apparently lay well. And so, the argument goes, they must be happy. What nonsense! Humans can co-habit and give birth in dungeons, but that doesn't make dungeons acceptable.

Leaving aside the emotional impact of all this on anyone who cares about cruelty to animals, how do the birds survive? The short answer is chemicals.

The poultry industry today is geared to mass production, but the factory farmers have run into two kinds of trouble: infection and behaviour disorders, which always occur when living creatures are jammed together in polluted enclosures.

Crowded indoors, without sun or contact with the soil, fed on processed foods containing pesticides and hormones, the birds succumb to disease unless heavily medicated with antibiotics. Without them too many birds would die. This was admitted back in 1960 at a US symposium on chemicals applied to soils, plants and animals.[13]

Antibiotics in poultry feed are also effective in hastening

weight gain in birds kept under crowded insanitary conditions, but their use encourages the growth of fungi and moulds in the intestines. So fungicides are added to the feed. A tranquillizing additive is also included to counteract stresses and tensions suffered by the birds – especially during hot weather, during handling for vaccination, de-beaking (to stop them pecking each other) and moving. Many of these chemicals cause dermatitis in poultrymen. Hormones have been used in poultry production even longer than in other livestock. For many years stilboestrol (female hormone) implants were used to caponize cockerels and fatten them cheaply. Then it was found that these hormone pellets were not always absorbed and that stilboestrol could induce cancer. Residue of hormonized chickens sold to mink farmers caused sterility in minks. Sex hormone implants are now used less extensively than they used to be.

At about this time, news that this female hormone was being put into chicken reached Italy – machismo among male Italians is strong and halted the Italian broiler industry. The import of sex-hormone-treated birds was stopped.

To sum up, the battery production of poultry for human food is unsatisfactory; not only is the taste of the meat and eggs from such birds inferior, but the chemical residues in them present a real threat to the health of susceptible people like Diana and David when they eat them.

It is time we stopped ignoring the nature of healthy chickens in our attempts to subjugate them to factory methods and learned to work with their biological needs so that they can live out their days in conditions suitable to their health as well as ours.

Factory-made convenience foods are processed, packaged, canned or frozen in order to stop them from going bad and to extend their shelf-life and out-of-season availability. They are becoming increasingly popular because they require less preparing and cooking in the home or canteen, which suits the housewife who goes out to work.

All convenience foods contain hidden ingredients which are a hazard to the food-allergic consumer. These hidden ingredients

are of two kinds: natural and synthetic, put there by the manufacturers.

Certain sugars, starches, oils, split protein products, gums,
alcohols and other derivatives of naturally occurring foods tend
to turn up with monotonous regularity in convenience meals
which also contain minute residues of chemicals used in production and processing. The synthetic ones are usually derived
from petroleum, coal tar or cellulose. These man-made chemicals
are added deliberately to make the product look, feel or taste
better, to retard spoilage or to simplify and cheapen manufacturing processes.

Clinical experience has incriminated these artificial additives
as causative agents in a wide range of behavioural problems,
hyperactivity and learning disorders, as well as in asthma,
urticaria, digestive disturbances and other allergic illnesses.
Lockey[30] and Randolph[42] both published papers on the subject
and since then many other investigators have published similar
findings.

It is not surprising that these additives and contaminants in
food and medicines should cause symptoms from adaptive overload in susceptible people, when you consider the amounts
ingested (three or four pounds per year per person) and their
almost limitless variety: bleaches, colours, flavourants, preservatives, thickeners, gums, buffers, acidulants, suspending
agents, texture modifiers, emulsifiers, surface-active agents,
chelating agents, anti-oxidants, anti-bacterials, anti-biotics,
mould-retarders, humectants (moisturizers), organic solvents,
enzymes, vitamins, minerals, alcohols (e.g. glycerol, sorbitol
and mannitol), sweeteners and flavour-potentiators including
sugar, saccharin, dextri-maltose, salt, monosodium glutamate,
nucleotides and citric acid. You need to be an industrial chemist
even to understand some of the names.

These added ingredients may be given on the label in vague
terms such as 'permitted antioxidant' or 'permitted colouring'.
Or, they may not be given at all. Labelling of food ingredients in
Britain and America is usually incomplete and frequently misleading, so that shopping in a supermarket for the person with

specific food and chemical sensitivities is like negotiating a minefield.

Among natural or source foods commonly included in convenience foods as labelled or unlabelled ingredients are egg, milk, wheat, soya, pork, beef, yeast, corn and peanut.

One little girl, whose bouts of abdominal colic I had managed to control by eliminating cereal grains from her diet, began to have colic again on what I and her mother thought was a strict cereal-exclusion diet. On a house call to the child in one of her attacks, I spotted a bottle of a well-known beef extract from which her mother had been making hot drinks. On reading the label I found that it contained wheat! Banning this tasty beverage resulted in no more colic.

For the milk-sensitive patient things can be difficult. Most 'non-dairy' products do contain such milk products as casein, caseinate, lactose and whey, and all of them contain ingredients from unexpected sources; corn, soya, beef, pork and lamb fat, vegetable oils and petrochemicals.

Powdered artificial sweeteners contain lactose (milk sugar) dextrose (corn sugar) as well as saccharin derived from coal tar.

Yeast, a potent sensitizer for many allergic people, is found in bakery products, alcoholic drinks, ketchup, mayonnaise and barbecue sauce, and in tea, the leaves of which are yeast-fermented, and other products enriched with yeast-derived B complex vitamins (including some packaged breakfast cereals).

It is inevitable that lubricating oils used on mixing, slicing and wrapping machinery used in food factories, should contaminate the food. So also will chemicals used to control bacteria, moulds, insects, rats and mice. While the amounts may not be above currently allowed toxicity levels, they are sufficient to cause allergic reactions in consumers sensitive to these chemicals.

So much for the chemical pollution of food, which affects nearly everything we eat. Now to consider indoor air pollution, the most insidious and hitherto least suspected factor in the epidemic of polysymptomatic disease now threatening urban man.

SEVEN

Gas and indoor air pollution

When I got my own practice in 1952, in Kew, long before I learned about clinical ecology, I persuaded two families plagued with repeated attacks of sore throats and bronchitis for whom drugs were doing nothing to move from damp houses near the river to drier places up on Richmond Hill. Something in those riverside houses – moulds probably – seemed to be keeping the occupants ill. After carrying out this simple though expensive manoeuvre on my recommendation, these patients were grateful to me in years to come.

It is no exaggeration to say that people take in greater quantities of harmful substances via their lungs than they ever do by mouth or through the skin. The absorbing area of the alveoli, the myriad air sacs in the lungs, is equal to that of a tennis court and a large proportion of chemicals which will evaporate such as paint, or floor and furniture polishes will end up inside the people breathing the air in the building.

The growing tendency for industry to offer chemical remedies for all sorts of household problems, from flies and cockroaches to bathroom and kitchen smells, is adding to the pollution hazards of indoor air, already troublesome to many people because of fumes from gas and oil-burning appliances.

It is difficult to imagine a more dangerous way of supplying energy for cooking, hot water and central heating than gas.

Hardly a day goes by without a report in the newspapers or on the radio that people have been killed or maimed in explosions involving domestic gas. I have a file full of such newspaper cuttings. One[9] shows a picture of a twenty-one-storey block of flats with smoke coming from the sixteenth floor. The caption reads, 'Smoke pouring yesterday from a tower block in Battersea, where a gas explosion killed one resident and left more than 100 families homeless after the building had been evacuated'. Think how much gas those families must have breathed into their lungs. You are not safe nowadays even in an all-electric house. Leaky old gas pipes may lie nearby.

Such deaths are the tragic price we must pay for having a relatively cheap source of energy piped into our houses. But what about susceptible people made chronically sick from exposure to gas fumes, burnt and unburnt, in places not in immediate danger from explosion: houses and offices heated by gas?

Soon after I had learned about chemical allergy from Dr Randolph, a patient consulted me about her depression. As there did not seem to be anything particularly depressing about her circumstances, or personal relationships with her family, I went to look at her house and on entering the front door noticed a faint smell of gas. She could smell it too and had already been on to the Gas Board who had sent workmen to locate the leak but could not find one.

She went on complaining and the Gas Board kept on sending people to inspect her house but without any result. Her depression continued. Eventually she and I combined to send a strongly worded letter, and a senior man came with two engineers. They removed the gas meter and dismantled it on the lawn. The leak was on the supplier's side of the meter. A new one was installed with new piping out to the main in the road and the smell ceased. Shortly after this, her depression cleared up as mysteriously as it had come on.

My patient was an educated, intelligent woman, married to a man in the film business and between them they decided to sue the Gas Board. Before the case came to court, the Board offered £350 (a fair sum in those days) with a 'no further responsibility' clause in settlement of the claim. This was accepted and the case closed.

Dr Randolph, who has had vastly greater experience of gas-sensitive patients than I have, published a paper on depression caused by gas, in 1955[43]. He gives more details of the problem in his book.[44]

Here are some relevant quotations from that book: 'Despite

the fact that utility gas is the cleanest of the readily available fuels, it is also the most hazardous for the majority of chemically susceptible patients. It seems to make little difference whether artificial or natural gas is used, although the relatively high pressures under which natural gas is currently delivered may increase this hazard, especially if home installations have been designed for lower pressures. As a consequence, every joint and turn in a utility gas line is a potential and oft-times an actual point of slight leakage. Utility gas, being lighter than air, tends to rise from the basement or kitchen through the remainder of the house.

'The greater the amount of piping and number of outlets, the more pilots and other automatic devices on gas utilities, the greater the potentiality and probability of leakage. Chronic symptoms may be maintained in the highly susceptible patient living in a gas utility home. This is due to leakage of unburned gas, even though all pilots are turned off, no gas is burned and despite the report of the Utility Company that gas leaks cannot be detected.'

When writing his book, he had already ordered the removal of over 500 gas-fired kitchen ranges from the homes of patients susceptible to chemical odours and fumes. 'One of the most amazing results of this experience,' he wrote, 'is that I have not received one major complaint from this group of patients regarding the expense of such a move. Once the indications for the move are present and the patient complies with the advice, resulting clinical improvement apparently has justified the expenditure.'

This evidence of the harmful effects on some susceptible people of repeatedly inhaling the burnt and unburnt fumes from domestic gas appliances must put in question the safety of anaesthetists, who spend long hours, day after day, inhaling small quantities of anaesthetic gasses in the operating theatre and anaesthetic room. It has long been known that anaesthetics are addictive and that some anaesthetists become so dependent on them that they disconnect the tubes from the gas cylinders, to take a quick drag to keep themselves 'topped up'. The alcoholic does the same if he has not had a drink for a certain length of time. This is the masking of allergic malaise by resort to the 'hair of the dog,' as described on page 82. This was elaborated in my paper on 'The Allergic Factor in Alcoholism'.[34]

In chapter three, Professor Rea described his own dizziness, headache and flu-like symptoms occuring in the operating theatre which required regular shots of dilute terpene extracts (basic petrochemicals from which anaesthetic gases are derived) in order to confer immunity and enable him to continue working as a surgeon.

So it could have been predicted that eventually anaesthetists themselves would study and report on the adverse effects of day-long exposure to anaesthetic gases. The *British Medical Journal* carried a paper by the Senior Lecturer[54] at Birmingham University's Department of Anaesthetics at Queen Elizabeth Hospital who had made a survey of all anaesthetists and their families in the West Midlands – one in ten of the 3400 anaesthetists in England and Wales. His findings confirm the worse fears of clinical ecologists:

> Thirty per cent of anaesthetists had problems in begetting children. Children born to hospital anaesthetists are sixty times more likely to suffer from cancer than other children. The incidence of breast cancer in women anaesthetists is fifty times higher than normal. Anaesthetists' children suffered a disproportionate number of neurological problems, sometimes severe. Three children died in infancy after convulsions and other manifestations of central nervous disturbance.

Medical officials at the Department of Health took the view that valid nationwide conclusions could not be drawn from the survey. A spokesman for the Health and Safety Committee said, 'We have been concerened about this problem for some time. We would like hospitals to get going on it.' Hospital administrators said they could not afford equipment to remove anaesthetic gas pollution from operating theatres.

Tragedies look different – according to where you are standing.

Clinical ecologists are all agreed that susceptibility to gas, oil and coal, including the combustion products and derivatives of these fossil fuels, is one of the commonest unsuspected causes of chronic illness. So common in fact, that simply moving a patient from a gas-fired house to an all-electric one may result in a gratifying reduction in the level of symptoms after a week or ten days.

One of my first chemical victim patients in the hospital, who suffered three or four epilepsy-like fits every day and who had baffled neurologists by becoming worse on anti-epileptic drugs, became free of fits when I arranged for her to go away to a gas-free house in the Scottish highlands. On returning home to her house in a Hampshire town where she cooked and heated by gas, her fits returned. Exposure to new paint or motor car exhausts aggravated her fits, as did foods containing chemical additives and the smell of newsprint. Anything derived from fossil fuels upset her.

As it was impossible for this girl to avoid inhaling gas and gas-related chemicals, her fits were eventually controlled with de-sensitizing sub-lingual drops of very dilute ethanol (synthetic alcohol 1:10,000) self-administered once or twice a day. This treatment is described more fully in chapter nine.

Dr Randolph states that indoor air pollution by gas and oil-burning appliances is of primary importance. It *must* be controlled before attempting to observe the clinical effects of exposure to other chemicals such as food additives, coal tar-related drugs, insecticides, alcohol, perfumes, bleaches, cigarette smoke and so on.

When a slightly susceptible person is first adapting to gas and gas-related chemicals, he tends to remain energetic and symptom-free so long as exposures to gas are frequent. He may even express a liking for gas and the odours of fresh paint and paraffin stoves. Only if he avoids these chemicals will he experience hang-over-like symptoms: headache, malaise, muscle aches etc., which clear after four or five days avoidance of gas (or sooner if masking occurs from re-exposure within two or three days).

But as adaptation to gas and everyday related chemicals decreases, characteristic overlapping and cumulative effects develop insidiously, so that neither the victims nor the doctor suspects their cause. Eventually, with progressive loss of adaptation, the victim is ill nearly all the time.

Randolph introduced me to a patient of his, a charming elderly lady, who allowed me to tape-record a talk with her. Here is an abbreviated version of that tape which illustrates how insidiously allergy to gas can affect people and the dramatic improvement which avoidance can bring about.

Dr Mac Can you describe how you felt before you consulted Dr Randolph and then tell me what happened.

Mrs D At that time my only trouble with allergies seemed to be first grass and then tree pollen in the spring. I was inoculated against them and it later hit me as hay fever in August and I would go away to try to avoid that and it was only a few years ago that this other trouble seemed to come on. I would note a little fluttering in my neck at odd times just like a pulse. If I were driving I would feel that I wanted to stop and wait. At this time I must have been in my late fifties or early sixties and I am now seventy-five.

Once I was in Chicago to attend a board meeting and I started to cross the street and I just started to have a little fluttery feeling and I went over and sat in our institute a little while and I thought it was nerves. It bothered me a little but I thought it might be – oh – palpitations, nervousness and I put it down a good deal to that. But that same kind of feeling became more noticeable and I got into this very serious phase of these symptoms. That was about eight or ten years ago.

Dr Mac What were these other symptoms?

Mrs D Dizziness and feeling I would pass out. I noted when I went down to buy my grandchildren some little gifts I would cling to a post before crossing at the light because I felt so frightened about getting to the other side, and yet nothing seemed to happen other than this sensation and I thought perhaps it was a form of nervous indigestion and that year I made my poor husband go out and buy 7 UP by the carton because I felt that would relieve the symptoms.

Dr Mac Did you drink a lot of 7 UP?

Mrs D I used to drink a lot of it, thinking that would relieve any pressure. It seemed that something of that sort would, but it didn't. Anyway, that year, when we got on the train to come home, we had this compartment and my husband asked me to come and look at this snow-covered mountain and I had to stoop and look up to see it from the other side of the compartment and just as I did that, I blacked out, and the next thing I knew, I was looking down at his wrist watch and I did not know what had happened but it frightened him terribly. 'When we get home,' he said, 'the first thing you are going to do is to go to the heart specialist and have a thorough going over.'

We heard of a very fine cardiologist, and we thought it would be good to start with him. I was very trembly in the hands, and this dizziness had increased. The specialist made two or three examinations and took an electro-cardiogram, said that I had a cardiac arrythmia and I believe gave me some little pills of belladona and I think it was at that time that he gave me also very minute doses of phenobarbitol. Then he suggested that I go for an examination to the hospital where I could have a thorough going over. He couldn't exactly diagnose from what he had observed, so I went into the hospital. They could not find anything and they had all these X-rays, GI tests and so on. They could find only that I had gallstones, not thinking that these were gallstone-caused symptoms. At least, they did not take them too seriously and by this time, it was about time for me to go north to avoid hay fever. Then I went to Dr Randolph for some hay fever shots and he felt my symptoms might be allergic ones, which he might be able to help with. He told me that I should keep a food diary and write down everything I ate so that he could go through my diet with me. But the hay fever season came on and it was time to go north and I went with my phenobarbitol etc., and the most I can remember that year was that my hands were very trembly and at times I was walking kind of dizzily and I remember walking down to the beach a number of times feeling as though I was lifting my feet maybe two feet high to take a step. I had the most peculiar sensation but since then I have found out that the cottage I occupied was heated with butane gas, and also the hotel manager used fly spray to clear the lobby at dinner time and one night after dinner, my sister was with me and I was looking at a map where we had been on the beach that day and I started to point out where we had been, and next thing I knew I was on the floor in a faint. Everybody was very much concerned and thought that I might not live till Christmas but I came home and fooled them. By the time I got home, my cardiology doctor found that I had lost so much weight that he wanted me to go back in the hospital; so within a year I had been in twice for almost a week each time, having every kind of test. They couldn't find anything to lay their finger on.

Very much mystified, I took my food diary to Dr Randolph and he saw that I had been having these sensations of blacking out after I had eaten quite a bit of Jello. He said, 'Jello has colouring matter in and if you react to that, you could be in the chemical field.' Then he asked me about my gas stove and I said yes I had one and he said, 'I think you should consider taking it out.'

Well, after that, I fell in the kitchen one day, getting breakfast and then my husband and I both knew that it must be the gas stove which was not well vented. Another doctor who had seen me at Dr Randolph's had urged me to take out the gas stove. He said that people who have allergies have trouble so often with chemicals and don't realize it is the gas. Both my husband and I had our doubts about it but we went ahead and got rid of the stove.

Dr Mac Do you feel well now?

Mrs D I feel really well indeed.

Dr Mac If you happen to eat Jello or go into gas, does it affect you?

Mrs D No, no, and I must say, I have been places where there is gas and it no longer affects me. I think Dr Randolph felt too, that this was just an overload that I had in my life at that time when I would come into contact with more than I could take.

Dr Mac   Do you notice any trouble from sprays?

Mrs D   Well, I notice more of a hay fever reaction to that, I have a cloudy voice and cough and blow my nose, but not dizziness.

I said I thought it was very good testimony and it clarified a number of things about chemical allergy which Ted Randolph had been telling me, e.g. the overlap between inhaled chemicals like gas and related coal tar-derived colourings in foods like Jello.

It also illustrated the barrel effect. Mrs D. did not have to avoid all her allergens completely to get well. We just had to remove her major allergic load which was domestic gas. Lowering the level of liquid in her barrel by turning off one of the most troublesome taps, reducing the strain on her powers of adaptation to the point where she could cope again with her physical environment without symptoms.

It is a lucky coincidence that medical realization of the hazards to health from domestic gas should be dawning just at the time when the world is being hit by a short-fall in supplies of fossil fuels, making them so expensive that safer alternatives such as wind, wave-power and solar, geothermal and nuclear energy are becoming economic alternatives worth researching and bringing into use to generate electricity.

That most intelligent and readable political commentator, Andrew Alexander, writing in the *Daily Mail* on 11 June 1979, has suggested seriously that Sir Geoffrey Howe, the new Conservative Chancellor of the Exchequer, should sell the British National Oil Corporation which supplies the country with gas and oil from the North Sea. 'It is a marvellous time to sell oil assets,' he wrote. 'One of the attractions of selling oil shareholdings is that it is easy to get foreigners to buy them. Thus the money comes from abroad to the Treasury and it does not affect the capacity of the British capital market to finance the

Government's and industry's requirements. It is hard to put a value on BNOC but by selling off most of BP and BNOC about £3 billion might be realized, perhaps more.' In his budget speech, Sir Geoffrey announced that he was selling part of the Government holding in BP. With a sum like that, industry could be encouraged to find cheap, abundant sources of electricity quickly. Within five years the gas taps could be turned off, petrol pumps closed down and our roads and railways converted totally to electric vehicles run on electricity or on hydrogen produced by electrolysis of water.

After a broadcast I did on the subject of food and chemical allergy on 31 May 1979, a woman wrote me a letter, part of which I quote, with her permission:

Dear Doctor,

Having heard you being interviewed on Radio 4 on Thursday morning last, about the current research into allergies, I feel prompted to write and give personal experience which might provide useful data to those engaged in the project.

The allergies from which I suffer are not connected with food, but smells. This trouble has worried me for some years but seems to be progressive as it is getting worse. Smoke, both from bonfires and tobacco, though the latter is the greater, result in a very sore throat. Fumes, let out into the atmosphere by gas and oil-fired central heating plants from quite a long distance away, give me nausea. Detergents, washing powders and air fresheners are among the worst offenders as they are so strongly scented. Also cleaning powders like Vim, containing bleach, as well as strong scents. Being unable to utilize such things makes life very difficult. There are *no* unscented washing powders or abrasives on the market and all the aforementioned products not only give me a sore throat but smarting eyes. I have had to give up having my straight hair permanently waved as the effect of the smell of the lotion on my eyes lasts for weeks. One of the worst deprivations resulting from the disability is that I cannot buy new clothes and have to walk around in coats and dresses purchased up to twelve or thirteen years ago because of the texturizing agent now used in the material.

If the research results in a general antidote, I should be very grateful to be informed.

My doctor in London said that all I could do was to try and avoid the smells which affected me most. But this is impossible. About an hour ago I became conscious of aerosol air freshener seeping into my flat round the cracks of the door and discovered that it was coming from the open door of the flat opposite me on the landing. So I opened my windows wide to let in as much fresh air as possible but had to close them straight away as cigarette smoke was rising up and coming in from the open window of the flat below. Such is life. 'Tween the devil and the deep sea!

EIGHT

Extending the ecological approach

Readers who have come this far will have gathered that clinical ecology is about patients who do not get well under the present system of medical practice. It offers them and their doctors a different way of looking at ill-health. Not a panacea – clinical ecology has its quota of failures – but an alternative approach, which offers hope where previously there was none.

Schizophrenia is a particularly appropriate illness to look at to see how clinical ecology might help when current treatments fail. The word schizophrenia, which means split or divided mind when literally translated, was coined in 1911 by the German psychiatrist, Eugen Bleuler to replace the earlier name 'dementia praecox' which meant premature loss of mental capacity.

The schizophrenic has not lost his mental capacity in the sense that a demented old person has. His thought processes are temporarily out of gear and he has developed a split or incongruity between feeling and the content of his thoughts. His emotional tone is flat and he may have delusions and hallucinations. It is a mysterious and insidious disease, tragic because it afflicts mainly young people in their late teens and early twenties. Despite certain differences in criteria for making the diagnosis, it is estimated that schizophrenia affects about one in every hundred of the population in Western countries. It is a colossal problem, and as with all illnesses of unknown cause, medical approaches to schizophrenia vary according to the type of knowledge to which the doctor subscribes.

The following case, sent to me by a mother whose son appeared to be developing schizophrenia, illustrates what can be done on ecological lines. I would emphasize that I never actually saw this boy. His mother had read *Not All in the Mind* and applied the methods described in it.

> 'My second son has never been as healthy as my eldest and youngest sons. He was always more susceptible to colds, catarrh, ear troubles, etc., as a child and was always, as the school said " in a permanent sort of daydream". He was always quiet, well behaved and no trouble, never going far from home and spending quite a lot of time on his own in his room.
>
> 'In the last two years, however, he had become increasingly susceptible to colds, headache-prone, anxious and always with indigestion, which in a boy of his age I knew not to be right.'

From her description of his symptoms, any psychiatrist who has watched the development of a full-blown schizophrenic illness in an adolescent would agree that this case must have looked ominous. The withdrawal, vagueness and perpetual irrational worrying are typical of early schizophrenia. The teenager who seems to be 'in a permanent sort of daydream' is always at risk.

> 'On a couple of occasions I had taken him to the doctor because of his general lethargy, lack of concentration and all the other symptoms. The doctor seemed to think it was all part of growing up and told me to let him have a few days off school and relax.
>
> 'He had been growing steadily worse, and was ending up not eating at all as he said that everything he ate made him feel better at first and then increasingly ill. At about this time he had a bout of "tummy trouble" and I had to keep him off food for three days to get rid of it. However, by the third day he said that he had never felt so well in his life! At this stage I felt I needed to find out if it was a type of food that was affecting him and very fortunately for us we found the book by Richard Mackarness. We did the tests on him one by one and there was absolutely no doubt about it any more. The food which was literally poisoning him was wheat in all forms, the very worst being white bread, pastry made with white flour, biscuits, etc. This was the type of food that he was always eating and having

snacks of. We have since found that he is sensitive to all grain, much less so to rice, but still with a certain reaction.

'He has now been off all grain for approximately four months and the change in him is staggering. He laughs, jokes, makes conversation, is interested in things and above all says that he no longer worries and worries over everything, whilst not really knowing what on earth he was worrying about. He says that until now he thought that everyone used to worry like he did, and he didn't know how they could take it. The most important thing is that he has now obtained an interesting job and is riding a powered cycle, two things which he simply would not have been able to do while on wheat because he was so absent-minded and forgetful.

'When I discovered that I had found the cause of his trouble I arranged to see a consultant about it. I thought perhaps he could help with diet but unfortunately he only talked about testing him for gluten reaction, so I cancelled the investigations and we dealt with it ourselves. He eats potato cakes at times when he would at other times have eaten bread, say with bacon and eggs for breakfast, and is able to eat all fish, meat, cheese, salads, veg. and some fruits. Food which makes him react, much less strongly than wheat, are strawberries and some citrus fruits.

'Of course, now that he is totally off wheat, if he makes a mistake like he did a little while ago and eats some flour in food accidentally, he reacts very strongly indeed, and I enclose a chart of what happened to him when he did this.

'My son has since said that he has never felt so carefree and optimistic. He never knew what it was not to feel worried and anxious and used to go into his room just to worry about things one after the other. At the time of course he never told me of these feelings, thinking that they were natural.

'He has been perfectly fit ever since coming off wheat, working from 8 a.m. to 5.30 p.m. on his feet all day and not having a single day off. (He was always home from school.)

'If any mother notices the same symptoms in her child I would strongly advise her to try these food tests. It has made

all the difference to my son's and my own life. Wheat was
poisoning him just as surely as cigarettes or drink would
another person.'

The changes in the size of the pupil, which the boy's mother
mentioned in her notes of his reaction to eating bread, is a
very important sign of brain involvement in an allergic reaction
to challenge with a food or chemical. It is evidence of changes in
nor-adrenalin and dopamine levels, two of the biochemical
transmitters of nerve impulses. Pharmaceutical companies, with
the help of reductionist psychiatrists, have studied these neurotransmitters intensively and have discovered drugs which will
oppose them when their levels in certain parts of the brain become too high. This has brought about a minor revolution in the
treatment of schizophrenia and manic depression (the two major
psychiatric illnesses), enabling many mental patients to leave
hospital and live some sort of life outside.

This type of biological and experimental approach to schizophrenia seems to me to be more likely to produce results than the
approach still being taken by official psychiatry in Britain and
America as typified frequently in the *British Journal of Psychiatry*
(laughingly referred to by its readers as the yellow peril because
of its vivid yellow cover).

The unspoken assumption is that schizophrenia is all in the
mind and we do not have to do more than describe what a
disordered mind seems to be doing to itself to call it research and
get a long paper published in a prestigious psychiatric journal.
Thought cannot occur without a brain. Healthy brains can think
normally. Unhealthy, allergic or poisoned brains think abnorm-
ally. Why? and what can be done about it?

These are the questions clinical ecologists and biochemists are
trying to answer. The answers are coming as a result of increasing
knowledge of the biochemistry and metabolism of the brain.
Passage of nerve impulses within the brain and along nerves takes
place by means of movement of chemical ions (electrically
charged chemical particles) across the membranes which divide
one nerve cell from another.

Food-derived glucose in the blood stream provides the energy for this, together with oxygen brought in from the lungs. Glucose can be made from fat, protein or carbohydrate in the diet. To obtain energy from glucose and oxygen requires enzymes (as catalysts) which oxidize the glucose to carbon dioxide and water. Petrochemicals and other toxic substances poison these enzyme systems and cause brain cell metabolism to become abnormal, leading to clinical depression and thought disorder.

Chemical transmitter systems in the brain are easily upset by allergy, malnutrition and toxic products of metabolism. Clean air, chemical-free water and simple organic food have always and will always provide the best context in which brain cells can work normally.

I am thankful to report that a lot of doctors and patients are becoming critical of the all-in-the-mind approach, and of the equally sterile Marxist myth beloved of social workers: that mental illness is the result of inequalities in the social system. Here is Dr Morton Sandler, distinguished biochemist at the Bernhard Baron Memorial Research Laboratories, Department of Clinical Pathology, Queen Charlotte's Hospital for Women, London, on the subject:[37]

'A generation ago it would have been unthinkable to attempt to define schizophrenia in terms of anything other than the somewhat mysterious psychological concepts of the time. This approach, which had little contact with everyday physical experience, produced theoretical constructs that were blinkered by their own limited set of assumptions. The major questions were pre-empted, the arguments were circular and scientifically no progress was possible.'

Well, progress is possible today. Not only in schizophrenia but in a whole range of mental and physical disorders still regarded as incurable and impossible to prevent. Viewed ecologically these mysterious disorders which compose our modern epidemics, can be tackled from a new angle. Some, like lung cancer, alcoholism and venereal disease, are already known to be ecological and capable of prevention by cutting off contact with the specific environmental factors; tobacco, intoxicating liquor, and the germs of sexually-transmitted infection. Economic and social considerations have obstructed effective measures of control, but at least the causes are known.

The link between lung cancer and cigarette smoking was established by a well-designed piece of prospective epidemiologica-research in 1950[12]. Alcoholism, now on the increase and estimated to be costing the British economy 500 to 1000 million pounds annually through inefficiency, sickness and absenteeism, has never been seen as anything other than a self-inflicted environmental disorder. Venereal disease, also on the increase, was shown to be environmental when Schaudin isolated the spirochaete causing syphilis in 1905.[50] Sir Alexander Fleming gave us an effective remedy in penicillin back in the 1930s but the permissive society has pushed the case load up so high that our modern pox doctors working from their discreetly named genito-urinary medicine clinics cannot chase up more than a fraction of the infected people.

These are diseases where a combination of common sense observation, epidemiology and reductionist research has established environmental causes. Political and social factors now stand in the way of their eradication, but at least the causes are known and remedies are available if we care to apply them. Not so with rheumatism, heart attacks and behaviour disorders. The millions and millions of pounds and dollars spent on reductionist research, drugs and the psycho-somatic approach have failed to make much headway against these, until quite recently when Clinical Ecology units began to offer new hope to sufferers, simply by separating them from specific foods and chemicals and showing that their symptoms can be reduced and brought back again on challenge with the avoided materials, thus demonstrating cause and effect.

At the South Eastern Chronic Disease Center in North Carolina, Dr Murray Carroll and his partner, Dr Thurmin Bullock, have reported on 316 cases of arthritis, studied over three-and-a-half years. Here is a summary of their findings[6]:

Prior to hospitalization, those patients who appeared to present with a hypersensitivity problem were evaluated in our office where an extensive history was taken. It became obvious that many patients with arthritis also had a history of other system complaints such as asthma, drug reactions, migraine headaches, chronic gastro-intestinal disorders, emotional instability or other manifestations which had not been previously diagnosed as being allergic and had been treated symptomatically. Therefore, particular emphasis was directed to possible past allergic symptoms.

Patients were taken into our county hospital. Since the inter-relationships of food, inhalant and chemical hypersensitivities remain to be fully explored we tried to make the environment of the unit as chemically clean as possible, so as to facilitate more accurate detection of food hypersensitivities.

Following the fast, which cleared the digestive tract and induced a hypersensitive state, food challenges were begun. Between forty and one hundred such challenges were done on each patient. Evaluation was by questionnaire and direct observation. The results were as follows:

	Diagnosis	*Yes*	*No*
Did the condition improve while in hospital?	Osteo-arthritis	98	2
	Rheumatoid	91	7
While eliminating allergenic foods, did the conditions remain improved after going home?	Osteo-arthritis	89	8
	Rheumatoid	81	19

Degree of improvement while avoiding allergenic foods	100%	50–99%	1–50%	0%
Osteoarthrisis	27%	52%	13%	7%
Rheumatoid arthritis	11%	46%	26%	17%

Foods incriminated, in order of frequency

Corn	37%	Pork	19%	Tomato	9%
Wheat	27%	Apples	14%	Butter	
Milk	23%	Cola	14%	beans	9%
Coffee	22%	Oranges	12%	Peanuts	8%
Tea	22%	Chocolate	11%		
Sugar	20%	Beef	9%		

These results warrant further examination by rheumatologists and already confirmation is coming in from other centres studying arthritis.

A criticism of this study is that it did not clearly distinguish between plain organic foods and commercial, chemically contaminated foods. Other doctors have now done this. Nevertheless, Carroll and Bullock's observations support the hypothesis that a direct correlation exists between the symptoms of rheumatism affecting the musculo-skeletal system and hypersensitivities to foods. This correlation has been reported by other clinical ecologists studying patients with symptoms involving other body systems.

The reason why more doctors have not yet found these correlations is that they have not looked for them. Recently, I was asked by Dr Judith Darmady, paediatrician at my hospital and one of the kindest and most human physicians I have ever met, to look at a twelve-year-old boy, Patrick, on the children's ward. He had giant urticaria (or hives), which brought him out in large itchy bumps, for no apparent reason.

Not knowing what else to do, Dr Darmady had proposed to put him on steroid drugs. I persuaded her not to, and put the boy on a Stone Age diet[32] (see also appendix E). This eliminated all the cakes, sweets and highly-coloured and flavoured drinks on which he was hooked, and the rash cleared up with no medication at all. Patrick was particularly fond of an artificial strawberry-flavoured syrup his mother used to put in his milkshakes.

Some weeks after he had gone home, still on the exclusion diet, Patrick suffered a minor injury and was brought to Accident/

Emergency, where, after exclusion of a fracture, he was given two aspirin tablets for his pain. Within a few minutes, his itchy bumps were back. Aspirin is a coal-tar derivative, as are many synthetic dyes used to colour foods and drinks. Coal-tar comes from the fossil fuel deposits which are one of the basic raw materials of the synthetic chemical industry. Patrick's allergy seems to be mainly to the artificial colourings in food, many of which contain tartrazine, an aspirin-related coal-tar compound.

Several allergists have reported adverse reactions to tartrazine in sensitive people. Dr Stephen Lockey[30] has found cases of generalized urticaria caused by tartrazine-containing foods and Dr Ben Feingold has attributed hives and swellings of blood vessels to tartrazine[14]. Randolph has reported extreme reactions in people sensitive to food dyes in imitation fruit drinks and alcoholic beverages. In one case a fifteen-year-old boy who did not react to chemically uncontaminated grapes, had an epileptic-like seizure after he drank an artificially coloured, grape-flavoured drink. Trial ingestion of the suspect dye precipitated a similar fit.[44]

Lockey reported two cases[31] where ice cream flavoured with artificial chocolate and artificial strawberry brought on anaphylactic shock. It seems that these tartrazine-based flavourings and dyes act as haptens which latch on to body proteins to form antigens which can precipitate severe reactions in sensitive individuals.

So, we are moving towards the conclusion that a lot of food allergy is really chemical allergy in disguise, and that many of the mysterious illnesses now taxing our health services are causally related to chemical pollution of food and indoor air. Which brings me to the modern captain of the men of death: coronorary thrombosis.

Professor William Rea was elected President of the International Society for Clinical Ecology for the year 1977/78 on the strength of the work he has done on environmentally triggered disease of the heart and blood vessels. The magnitude of his contribution to our understanding of this problem is not yet widely appreciated but I predict that it soon will be. He has shown that susceptible patients can react to inhaled chemicals within the first ninety minutes of being given a dose and that after-effects last up to forty-eight hours. Patients reacted to the fumes of the flame of a gas pilot light showing assorted symptoms, amongst them cardiac distress.

Much has been written recently about ill effects of aerosols and glue sniffing. Taylor and Hern[52] reported the death from heart failure of a sixteen-year-old boy following addictive sniffing of an aerosol, containing petrochemical fluorocarbon propellant, and there has been a report of inflammatory changes in the hearts and blood vessels of sea animals exposed to oil spills.

In June 1979, after a fifteen-year-old boy was found dead from glue-sniffing in the playing fields of a London school, the Hornsey Coroner, Dr David Paul, warned that the practice of sniffing chemical substances is 'as infectious as measles' and that it was most unlikely that the incident was isolated. A bottle found near the dead boy contained sixteen different compounds including paraffins and other hydrocarbons, fifteen of which were found in his blood post-mortem. The cause of death was given by the pathologist as plastic bag asphyxia precipitated by the inhalation of volatile substances.

Many glue-sniffers adopt the dangerous practice of putting a plastic bag over their heads to concentrate the volatile substances being inhaled and thus induce intoxication more quickly. Apart from the glue sold to stick model kits together, from which glue-sniffing gets its name, the substances sniffed include many in common domestic use: anti-freeze, coldstart, petrol, paint-thinner and stripper, lighter fuel, dry-cleaning fluids, hair lacquer and other aerosol sprays. The practice should more correctly be termed hydrocarbon or solvent inhalation, because volatile hydrocarbons are the main constituents of the substances sniffed or inhaled.

In the main, sniffing is a group activity. Lone sniffers usually have psychiatric problems associated with disturbed home backgrounds and in an attempt to escape unpleasant reality glue-sniffing becomes a habit. Stages in solvent addiction follow the familiar pattern of other addictions; with habituation in stage 2 (when large doses can be tolerated and sudden withdrawal causes 'shakes' and delirium), followed by resort to larger and larger doses to obtain the 'high' effect as the exhausted stage 3 is approached. The symptoms of overdose consist of initial excitement and inebriation, (sometimes with hallucinations) – the 'high' or 'buzz' sought by the addict – followed by progressive central nervous system depression ending in coma and death with very large doses.

Physical effects of long-term intermittent hydrocarbon inhalation include haematuria (blood in the urine from kidney damage), liver poisoning, anaemia and brain damage. Abnormal behaviour and even psychosis (insanity) can occur quite early in solvent addiction.

With our environment becoming steadily more contaminated with synthetic derivatives of petroleum-derived hydrocarbons it is important to realize how commonly these chemicals can induce disease in susceptible people.

The ill-effects of the chemical environment are lessened by showing patients how to avoid unnecessary exposure to chemicals. Symptoms will subside if a clean oasis can be created in one room at home – preferably the bedroom.

Compared with Dr Rea's set-up in his forty-bed Environmental Control Unit in Dallas, the arrangements for treating food and chemical-sensitive patients in my unit at Basingstoke are primitive. I am making do with a one-day-per week outpatient clinic and a sideroom here and there on the hospital wards, trying to keep them chemically clean with a notice on the door reading:

NO SPRAYS NO POLISHES PLEASE

I would dearly like to have a purpose-built ecological unit with ten or twelve beds and a day patient area. But that is unlikely at the moment, and I find there are certain advantages in being able to treat patients in a 1500 bed multi-department hospital. Other facilities not found in a small ecology unit are available.

Before the Psychiatric Intensive Care Unit in Basingstoke was shut down because the high ratio of staff to patients was judged to be too expensive, I was able to treat very disturbed patients in there and keep some control over their smoking and food intake. The few schizophrenics I have been able to get well on an ecological programme have relapsed since going home because once they slip off their strict exclusion diet, they become psychotic again and are very difficult to put back on the rails. Manic depressives have done a little better. But my best successes have been with patients who have a symptom which qualifies them for a bed on the medical floor, with or without mental symptoms. There, the facilities are good and patients have done very well indeed. One girl with ulcerative colitis who went temporarily mad, not only recovered her sanity but has also retained her colon and learned how to eat and structure her home environment so as to keep her diarrhoea, bleeding and abdominal pain away. Children are rewarding too. It is frustrating with psychiatric cases, to know that they could be helped, but not to have the staff or facilities to do anything effective.

Even so, I can take comfort from the patients who have improved, as readers will appreciate, if they turn back to the beginning of chapter one and re-read Loretta's case history. We'll now look at her case further.

When Loretta was due to have her baby in the Maternity Division, I thought that she would come unstuck, but the staff were so co-operative that all went well, in spite of the understandable apprehension expressed in this letter which she sent me on 7 June 1978:

Dear Dr Mac,

I would like to take you up on your offer to help me when I go into the 'Mini' (the name of the Maternity Unit) to have my baby on 25 July or thereabouts. I do not seem to be getting anywhere with the doctors and I think I am going to need a hand.

My general practitioner thinks that 'all this allergy business is nonsense' and gets very vague when I try to pin him down. Mr Payne is the consultant, and when I last saw him in March he seemed reasonable but on my last visit I saw another doctor and it appears that I will not be seeing Mr Payne again. The doctor I saw on my last ante-natal visit, on hearing my requests said that no special provisions will be made and that anyway 'surely it wouldn't matter for a week'. I need to know that the Maternity Unit is expecting someone who cannot eat certain foods. I am sure that I shall not be able to explain the problem properly while I'm in labour.

As I am also allergic to aerosol sprays, polishes, etc. I can foresee certain problems. I am not sure if anything can be done to help me there, at least if the staff know that I might be ill it will be a help.

The last thing that is worrying me is the possibility that my baby will be allergic. I have been told that if he cries during the night the staff will give him sugar and water; I don't know if this will be white sugar which will not be ok if the baby has inherited my allergies.

Every time that I have tried to clear up these problems, I have met vague looks and raised eyebrows with mutters about 'over-anxious pregnant women'.

I would be very grateful if you could help me with these problems. To remind you – I am allergic to white flour, milk and sugar. The food does not have as strong an effect as aerosol sprays, gas, polish and any other breathable chemicals.

I am planning to be at the Chemical Victims meeting on the 16th of June but I thought you would be too busy to talk about this.

Thank you.
    Loretta.

Loretta's experience is not unique. Many of my patients have run into similar difficulties when turning to other doctors for help along the lines I have taught them to follow and which they know from experience have kept them well.

In fact I told Dr Pugh, the South African registrar who worked for Mr Payne, the consultant obstetrician, about Loretta's problem. He was most helpful and suggested I tell Mrs Morrison, the Senior Nursing Officer in charge of the Maternity Unit. So

I did that, and went to see the dietician. The final hurdle was to get a single room allocated to Loretta and to persuade the cleaners not to spray her room with aerosols and to use no polish on her floor. Smoking is already banned in the Maternity Unit so that was not the problem that it is in the Psychiatric Division, where patients are encouraged to smoke at all times and in most places (except in bed) and where, as in prison, tobacco is the main currency and where the gift of a cigarette is often better than a tranquillizer pill for keeping a troublesome patient quiet.

After she had had her baby, Loretta sent me this further letter:

... I was admitted on Monday 31 July with a view to induction on Tuesday 1 August. Everyone knew I was the 'allergic one'. A notice saying 'Do not clean this room before consulting Sister' was put on the door of my room and two student nurses sat for half an hour asking about allergies. Breakfast was haddock (ok) white roll, butter, marmalade, oat crunchies, milk, sugar (not ok). However, the Sister soon sorted it out and some cheese was sent up.

Since then, after a chat with the sisters, nursing officers, Dr Brough, the house surgeon, and the dietician, and you of course, I have marked my menu with the food I can eat (nearly always salad) made up into a dish i.e. with cold meat or something ok. When there wasn't meat or fish I supplemented my food with fruit and 100% wholemeal bread and margarine brought in by Arthur.

I have used the loo and stayed in my room and for the first five days have remained completely free of any symptoms.

On day six, I was weepy (post-natal depression) and lonely and took a walk up to see my friend in one of the wards and stayed for a chat for ten minutes or so. Later a small rash developed. It soon went though. Served me right!

As for Andrew (the baby) he had dextrose for the first couple of days – I wasn't given the choice and I was too drugged after the delivery to think of it. Anyway I fed him fairly easily from the first. When he was 'topped up' with dextrose I could tell he didn't like it and on day three he had a rash so I said 'no more'. I topped him up with water and the rash went.

Since then, I have fully breast fed him, it means feeding him every three hours, but it is suiting him.

The only trouble over this was when a sister told me that he wasn't getting enough to eat. She said that I should be supplementing his breast milk with Ostermilk and that if I insisted on breast milk only, then I ought to make a better job of it.

Later that day, we weighed Andrew and found he had gained six ounces in twenty four hours – so I wasn't doing too bad a job!

Apart from that – everyone has been most particular about the cleaning.

I would like to say thank you as I know that it is due to your groundwork.

Loretta

Before she went home on the tenth day, the pathology laboratory reported her to be mildly anaemic with a haemoglobin level of 9.7 gms per dl (normal range in women who have just given birth: 10.5–15.0). It was suggested that she should be given iron by mouth, but as most iron preparations contain sugar I vetoed this and encouraged her to eat lots of meat and liver and to take sea salt for its content of trace elements (copper, iron, manganese, zinc etc.) which helps in making new blood.

She seemed happy with this and a further blood count in three weeks showed she was back to normal. Since then she and the baby have remained well and he is a fine boy.

After Loretta, who was the first to have an ecological baby in our maternity division, two other Chemical Victims Club members have had babies there and the routine has got well established.

To help these mothers bring up their children with minimal risk of allergy, I have been giving them a modification of a talk given by Edward Binkley, Jr, MD, now Medical Officer on the island of Guam, on 29 October 1977 at the Eleventh Advanced Seminar in Clinical Ecology in San Francisco.

Dr Binkley was President of the Society in 1974 and received the Jonathan Forman medal in 1978, for his work on the ecology of the unborn child and infant feeding.

Seeing many children who are hyperactive and who have behaviour disorders, learning disorders and multiple minor congenital anomalies led us to ponder the differences in the living conditions now and the living conditions twenty-five years ago. We then endeavoured to formulate a programme which would return the expectant mother as nearly as possible to pre-Second World War conditions.

The differences which were felt significant were the air inside and outside the home, water and food pollution, increase in radiation and consumption of empty calorie foods and 'junk' foods.

We then looked for some families who had children with minimal brain damage and who were going to have more children or where the mother was in early pregnancy. With their co-operation we changed the living conditions markedly as follows:

1 Both parents must stop smoking immediately.

2 No gas cooking stoves to be used.

3 Electric heat and/or hot water heat used if possible. A new all-electric home purchased, if feasible. If the home has forced air heating, the bedroom blowers are sealed off and a portable electric heater used (preferably the four-foot one made by Intertherm or King). The bedroom temperature reduced to below 20°C (68°F) in the winter to reduce the dust in the air.

4 If in an apartment, they should be on the highest floor possible.

5 No medication taken unless urgently needed. No aspirin.

6 No x-rays taken unless urgently needed.

7 The mother should not drink any alcoholic beverages.

8 No spray cans for any purpose allowed in the home.

9 No painting or decorating of the home is allowed.

10 Cleaning materials limited to plain soap for the laundry, bath and dishes. Washing soda or Borax allowed. Only unchlorinated scouring compounds allowed.

11 Cosmetics except for lipstick not allowed. Non-odorous deodorants used. Only cold water for after-shave treatment for the husband. Tooth powder to be made up of two parts salt and one part baking soda, powdered in a blender. A couple of drops of pure oil of peppermint added for flavour.

12 The diet limited to pure, plain foods without spices or herbs. Junk foods eliminated. Organic foods used if possible. Diet consisting mainly of meats, fruits, vegetables, spring water and sea salt. If possible, foods should be fresh, the frozen foods next, but not those contained in plastic bags. Canned or dried foods not advocated.

13 Childbirth without medication strived for.

14 Exercise during pregnancy strongly advised. Walking, bike riding, etc. are suggested.

15 Breast feeding of the newborn is insisted upon.

16 Allergies in the mother treated throughout pregnancy and during the period of breast feeding.

17 No hexachlorophene.

This programme, though strict, has resulted in progeny who are much less afflicted than older siblings.

Infant Feeding
Newborn Period – WATER only if something is needed. Not honey or glucose water. Honey sold in the shops is often diluted or cut with water and/or corn syrup. Therefore, get honey from a beekeeper or a health food store which certifies it to be pure and undiluted. Use in place of sugar. *Breast milk* if at all possible.

Two Months or Ten Pounds (later if not too hungry) – Vegetables on a three-day rotation (a food is used once only every third day). Carrots, marrow and peas. Later beans, spinach, beets or sweet potatoes. ALWAYS ROTATE. Use a spoon. Freeze unused portions.

Three Months – Fruits on a three-day rotation. Bananas, apples, peaches. Bananas are used fresh only. One-fourth banana is baked for fifteen minutes at 350°F. The banana is peeled first. Later fruits *other than* citrus can be added. ALWAYS ROTATE ALL FOODS. Use a spoon.

Four Months – Meats on a three-day rotation. Beef, pork and lamb. Later fish, sea foods and fowl. Meats are *plain*. They can be mixed with fruits or vegetables.

Five or Six Months – Cereals, pure, may have to be ground, mashed, blended or cooked. Commercial infant cereals have yeast in them. The more pure cereals are: Quaker Oats, plain brown rice, corn meal, millet cereal from the health food stores, or buckwheat. Use three or more on a three-day rotation or even a four or five-day rotation.

Six Months – Three meals per day with only water between meals.

Seven or Eight Months – Potato is added once every three days.

One Year – Citrus and egg are added for the first time to the diet and on a three-day rotation.

The three-day rotation diet is continued for as long as possible in the growing child.

NINE

Chemical victims of industry

Beware the humble carrot. It contains carratatoxin, a potent nerve poison. Not to mention myristicin, a hallucinogen wholly inappropriate for food. It also has isoflavines which imitate female sex hormones.

Radishes are not much better: they contain two substances which promote goitre by interfering with our uptake of iodine. Onions, olives, melons, potatoes and many other natural foods contain similar harmful substances. Fish has 40–170 parts per million of arsenic.

Guess who is giving this catalogue of gruesome ingredients? Not Dr Magnus Pyke. Not Ralph Nader, nor any ecology freak. It is Mr Stanley Freedman, Managing Director of McCormick Foods (UK) an American-based multi-national company, addressing the National Conference of the Food Manufacturers' Federation in London on Thursday 15 March 1979.

He was trying to show that if food safety standards imposed on man-made products were applied to natural foods, there would be hardly anything left to eat. He went on to say that various public paranoias about food safety differed in detailed symptoms, but all shared a common pathology (he was strong on medical jargon).

I admit he has got a point and I don't blame him for trying to discredit those who seek to restrict food manufacturers like his company from adulterating their products with more and more chemicals. But his arguments are irrelevant to the central ecological problem of our time: how are we to live and stay healthy in the chemical environment which he and the chemical conglomerates have created?

Most of us have inherited powers of adaptation equal to coping with mini-doses of poisons in the natural fruits and vegetables

on which we have evolved. But if he is right to warn us against
them, then surely this is an argument against putting *more*
chemicals in artificially, not a reason for knocking the existing
safety regulations and those who want to see them tightened
up.

Drug manufacturers use the same kind of ploy and say that
if we want new medicines we should let them put them on the
market without requiring too time-consuming and expensive tests
for safety. But we had the thalidomide tragedy. As recently as
1970, because tests were inadequate, practolol (Eraldin) was
allowed on to the market for the treatment of angina, high blood
pressure and disordered heart rhythm. It spite of being given the
all-clear by the UK Committee on Safety of Medicines, it killed
some patients by causing intestinal obstruction and made others
blind, before its prescription was restricted and ICI (the manufacturers) agreed to compensate 300 of the 1,000 people who
claimed to have been harmed by it.

Advocates of the highly dangerous nuclear power programmes
in Britain, France and America are also keen to be free of what
they see as petty restrictions on their activities and seek to discredit ecologists like Jacques Cousteau who lobby against them
on behalf of the lobster fishermen at Cap de La Hague, the people
living near Windscale and in Pennsylvania around the Three Mile
Island Atomic Power Station on the Susquehanna River in
America. Yet we know what happened to the people of Hiroshima, and radioactive hydrogen gas leaked dangerously at
Three Mile Island in April last year where Federal and State
officials had to evacuate pregnant women and children under
school age living within five miles of the crippled plant and make
plans to move a further 950,000 people from the four counties
of York, Lancaster, Cumberland and Dauphin.

Just as thalidomide made people uneasy about the drug
industry, so public suspicion of nuclear power will never be
dispelled after the crisis at Three Mile Island and the recent
reports of a leak at Windscale.

A similar no knowledge–no plans crisis is building up for
many susceptible people in respect to the chemical pollution of

food and drink. Clinical ecologists have good reason to be worried about what the food and chemical industries are doing to the environment, for as with radiation and drugs, events are proving the ecologists right. Disaster has actually overtaken some unlucky people as a result of commercial practices involving toxic chemicals.

In Michigan in 1974, a young dairy farmer found more and more of his calves born dead. Others died soon after birth. Cows lost their hair and grew hooves which curved upwards like mandarins' slippers. They staggered, wasted away and died. He was conscientious and it hurt when they told him he was not treating his cattle well.

Many specimens were sent for analysis to the laboratories in Michigan and neighbouring Maryland. Eventually, evidence was found of 400 to 4,000 parts per million of Firemaster, a newly introduced polybrominated biphenyl fire-retardant compound (PBB) in the bodies of the dead animals.

There had been a shortage of paper bags at the Firemaster factory and temporary brown bags had been used. One of these had got mixed in transit with similar-looking brown paper bags of magnesium oxide food supplement sent to the food preparation company.

Dead cattle were recycled and added to farm feed. By 1976, with farm products (milk, meat, eggs, cheese, etc.) contaminated, virtually the entire population of Michigan had PBB in their tissues.

Farmers became ill and sleepy. They were irritable and could no longer lift weights of more than fifty pounds. Professor Irving J. Selikoff and his colleagues of the Environmental Sciences Laboratory of the Mount Sinai School of Medicine undertook a survey of over a thousand dairy farm residents and people who had bought food from these farms, and found many of them ill, generally with measurable amounts of PBB in their body fat.

Fortunately, very little of this contaminated food was exported out of Michigan across state lines, since Michigan imports such food. If the same sequence of events had occurred in more prosperous neighbouring Wisconsin, which exports farm products, the whole of the United States could have been involved in the disaster.

The halogenated hydrocarbon compounds to which PBB belongs and which include chlordlane, aldrin, dieldrin, eldrin, lindane and DDT can easily get into food. They are used as wood preservatives and insecticides and are sometimes added to lubricating oils. They have killed dogs, cats and budgerigars housed in wooden sheds painted the year before, and have poisoned cattle eating hay stored in preserved wood sheds or grazing in fields crossed by preserved wood posts carrying electric cables.

Calves are very susceptible to halogenated hydrocarbons and succumb to skin, liver and nervous system disorders because the vitamin A is destroyed. Crumbs contaminated with oil with PCB from bread slicing machines have killed farm animals.[18]

The number of new agricultural sprays and granular chemicals being brought on to the market is now so great, that farmers now rely on the advice of the chemical companies' representatives to know when and how much a chemical needs to be applied to a growing crop. The implications for the consumer are frightening. Timing of applications must be exact; overdosing produces deformity and deficiency.

The chemical destruction of weeds on farms and in gardens has become so commonplace that nobody now thinks of the potential dangers to human health involved in spraying these biocides across the countryside from helicopters, tractor-drawn dispensers and small scale garden distributors.

Perhaps one of the most widely used selective weedkillers is 2–4.D (2–4 dichlorophenoxyacetic acid). This chemical is a synthetic growth regulator or 'plant hormone' which causes plants to overgrow and suffer fatal gigantism, so that they fall over and die. It has a most penetrating, unpleasant smell which has now replaced the pleasant greenhouse smell in garden shops with a nasty, chemical odour upsetting to many people. My wife is made quite ill by it and my next door neighbour, a keen gardener, has to go indoors and shut all her doors and windows when 2–4.D is being sprayed nearby, it makes her feel so ill.

Published reports on the toxicity of 2–4.D are scant but orally in animals it has not been shown to cause cancer or impair reproduction. By injection and after absorption through the skin it causes crippling and painful peripheral neuritis and there is an account of one housewife still severely incapacitated with neuritis after spraying the dandelions on her lawn with 2–4.D.

In summer 1978 there was a noticeable increase in fungus diseases on the wheat crop in Britian, reducing the yield by one quarter in certain areas.

Fungus disease on wheat can mean fungus in bread, unless the grain is properly dried. There is always a danger that fungi will grow and produce toxins (mycotoxins) which cause human disease. So wheat must be sprayed with fungicide to prevent the spread of fungus diseases.

Some of the Ministry of Agriculture's new high-yield bread wheats are particularly vulnerable to fungus. High-yielding seeds need a lot of ammonium nitrate. About one million tons of nitrate are spread on the land each year. But research in New Zealand has shown, unofficially, that high concentration of nitrate encourages the spread of fungus disease not only on wheat but in trees, perhaps causing Dutch elm disease and the diseases now starting to attack beech, ash and sycamore.

Nitrates can also cause disease in humans if too much runs off the land into the water supply. On several occasions the level of nitrates in London's drinking water has exceeded the safety limits recommended by the World Health Organization. But according to the Thames Water Authority this is not a matter for concern because it can be dealt with in future by adding another chemical to the drinking water.

Two stories of alarming effects of high nitrogen levels in water have made the news recently. During the long drought in Britain in 1976, drinking water evaporated from the reservoirs, concentrating the nitrates and other chemicals in the water that remained, to the point where it was unsafe to make up baby's bottles with tap water. In Norfolk, where the problem was particularly serious, special low-nitrate water had to be supplied to mothers of young babies.

In Chicago in 1963, there were notices all along the shores of Lake Michigan saying it was dangerous to swim in the water. Asking why, I was told that the lake had become poisonous from pollution with nitrates and industrial effluent. Apparently all the fish had been poisoned and the bottom of the lake was inhabited by millions of lampreys, primitive worm-like creatures resistant to pollution and parasitic on dead and dying fish. Public health experts feared that when these lampreys ran out of food, they too would die and rise to the surface as a rotting, stinking lake-wide raft. It hasn't happened yet, but it may do unless the lamp- reys learn to eat each other until there are none left.

The chemical industry, like the nuclear power industry, produces some very toxic products, by-products and waste, all of which have to be transported and disposed of. The driver of the bulk transporter of corrosive or inflammable chemicals may overturn his vehicle, killing and maiming innocent people, as happened in Spain recently, when a tanker full of liquid butane ran off the road, caught fire and burned alive people on a camping site.

In the East End of London, spillage from a formaldehyde tanker put forty-one people in hospital.

In 1977 the biocide plant at Seveso in Northern Italy which was making polychlorinated biphenyl (PCB) exploded. 1 kilogram- me of trichlorphenol was carried on the prevailing wind north of Milan. Thousands of people inhaled it. Birds and rabbits died. Men, women and children got sick.

Some PCBs such as the herbicides 2–4.D and 2–4–5.T, are poisonous. They can damage embryos at one part per trillion, causing multi-tissue tumours known as teratomas. No one knew what advice to give the Italians. In October 1979, the Ecology Party in Britain asked for an inquiry into the use of 2–4–5.T by the Forestry Department, claiming that it caused women to abort.

PCBs were used for defoliation in Vietnam and are extra- ordinarily persistent. They do not lose their toxicity for a long time. A German factory making PCB was closed after an ex- plosion; years later, a man dismantling the factory died of pancreatic failure and a child who used one of his towels died also.

In Japan, PCB leaked into rice oil, later used for cooking; babies were born brown, others were stillborn or deformed. People developed neurological disorders. Fish in the Hudson River, New York, contain PCB traced back to the dumping of PCB by the electrical industry. When PCB gets into breast milk, babies have all kinds of trouble affecting the skin and the nervous system. The catalogue of people damaged by chlorinated hydrocarbons goes on and on.

But that is only half the story. The other big group of toxic chemicals sold for use in the office, factory and home, as well as on the farm, are the organophosphorus insecticides. They are on sale without restriction in your local garden centre and hardware store. They include malathion, parathion, phosdrin, diazinon and TEPP. They contaminate vegetable produce, tobacco and the air inside cinemas, store-rooms, hotels and anywhere else they are sprayed.

These outstandingly dangerous compounds were first synthesized by German chemists in the 1930s and developed into potent nerve gases in preparation for the last war, but were never actually used in combat. After the war, many more were developed for use against aphids and other insect pests, as crop sprays and dusting powders for use by farmers and horticulturists.

Although one hundred times less toxic than the nerve gases from which they came, these organophosphorus compounds are still very toxic indeed. A one-milligramme dose is fatal, death occurring from respiratory failure. Signs of poisoning are: contracted pupils, tears, runny nose, drooling from the mouth, tight chest, laboured breathing, slow heartbeat, tremor, muscular twitching, gastro-intestinal disturbance, involuntary urination and defaecation.

Successful treatment depends on getting to the victim early and giving the antidote, atropine or oxine by injection. Soldiers are trained to recognize the symptoms and are issued with self-injection devices, when chemical weapons are expected to be encountered in combat.

A victim of organo-phosphorus poisoning can tolerate a two-milligramme dose of atropine by injection. The Army issues soldiers with three syringes, each carrying 2 mg. If the first injection is not enough, the second is given in fifteen minutes and the third fifteen minutes later. This level of dosage with atropine will cause dry mouth and dilated pupils.

In an emergency, civilians poisoned in the field should chew the berries and leaves of deadly nightshade (Atropa belladonna) which contain atropine. Chewing should be continued until symptoms of poisoning start to subside.

The basic pharmacology of all this is fairly simple: nerve impulses in certain parts of the brain and peripheral nervous system are transmitted from one neurone (nerve cell) to another by a chemical known as acetylcholine. This compound is secreted from the end of one neurone and crosses the gap to the next one to pass on the electrical impulse. In other words, acetylcholine is a neuro-transmitter substance, it acts on the parasympathetic nerves (which oppose the sympathetic nerves concerned in flight or fight and which run on adrenalin). If acetylcholine accumulates in the gap between one neuron and the next, it can over-stimulate the whole parasympathetic system (causing heart to slow, bowels to move, etc.) so, normally, there is an enzyme, cholinesterase, which clears the acetylcholine away once the nerve has 'fired'. *Organophosphorous nerve gases and pesticides destroy cholinesterase.* So the acetycholine piles up. The parasympathetic nervous system overacts, producing all the symptoms listed above. The atropine in belladonna opposes the action of acetylcholine and acts as an antidote.

This single cause–single antidote thinking is a bit limited when we are trying to deal with the wholesale slow poisoning of multiple enzyme systems occurring as a result of universal pollution of air, food and water with petrochemicals.

The key to our life processes is enzymes*. Most chemical reactions in the body are regulated by the catalytic action of enzymes, which are highly specific in their actions and each will only catalyse a small range of chemical transformations within

*The word means 'in yeast'. Louis Pasteur found that the fermentation of grape juice into wine was brought about by something in the yeast mould on the skin of the grape.

the living cells of which we are composed. If the integrity of enzymes is disturbed, then their catalytic power drops and you feel tired and ill.

Food and chemical allergy disturb enzyme systems in various ways, as does poisoning, as we have seen in the case of nerve gases and pesticides; the difference is only in the time scale: chronic effects with day after day exposure to allergens; immediate effects with poisons.

Now it is clear why organic pesticide-free food is good for allergic people. Clinical ecologists who prescribe compatible food instead of drugs are trying to preserve and restore enzyme systems.

A healthy, living human cell can conduct hundreds of simultaneous chemical reactions, each specifically catalysed by a different set of enzymes. These miraculous, interlocking and self-adjusting enzymes are all proteins and account for most of the protein content of the cell.

Consideration of these facts must make us question the wisdom of putting anti-enzymes into bread and spraying them on vegetables and fruit. They may retard moulds and kill aphids but they are also helping to kill us.

Although mainly composed of proteins, enzymes also require certain vitamins and minerals before they can function. Since the body can only get these from food it is dangerous to spray crops, while they are growing, with chemicals which interfere with the plants' uptake of minerals from the soil. Refining and processing plant foods like grain and fruit strips them of most of their vitamins; so people eating factory-produced food processed from sprayed crops are likely to end up enzyme-deficient. Orthomolecular treatment (see page 154) seeks to make good such deficiency by supplying the missing vitamins and minerals in pill and powder form, but such replacement therapy is expensive and slow to take effect.

As that great and wise physician Rene Dubois said, 'Men are naturally most impressed by diseases which have obvious manifestations, yet some of their worst enemies creep up on them unobtrusively.'

TEN

Questions and answers

This final chapter sums up the plight of the chemical victim in question and answer form, and tells how clinical ecology can help. Charts and tables referred to are in the appendix. *Before trying to treat yourself, please check with your doctor that you have not got something wrong with you that he can deal with or which should be referred to a specialist.* Many of the questions are those put by patients in my clinic or at meetings of the Chemical Victims Club.

Q   What is a chemical victim?
A   Someone whose health is being adversely affected by the modern chemical environment, by which I mean the substances in food, drinks, the air we breathe or things that touch us; these chemicals may be naturally occurring or, more likely, man-made. Some may be so toxic that everyone exposed to them becomes ill as in a pesticide factory disaster, or when food is contaminated with the toxin of botulism. These poisonous effects are obvious and can to some extent be guarded against by taking safety precautions.

More widespread and insidious effects come from allergy or hypersensitivity to substances which the majority of people seem to tolerate well. The chemical victim's allergy is a failure of adaptation to something with which his body is poorly equipped to deal, because of an enzyme defect or quirk of biochemical individuality, determined by inheritance.

Q   How does the illness show and what are the symptoms?
A   The symptoms are nearly always multiple and depend on the target organs or tissues affected by the allergy. Well-recognized targets are the nose and throat (as in hay fever or allergic rhinitis) the lungs (allergic asthma) and the skin (urticaria or hives).

Much less well recognized as allergic, but no less common, are migraine, disordered heart rhythm, indigestion, diarrhoea, weak bladder, muscle and joint pain, depression, agitation, anxiety, insomnia and the tension/fatigue syndrome. For a full list see appendix A.

Q But these conditions you have mentioned can have other causes. Surely they are not all allergic?

A Certainly they are not. They can be due to poisoning, infection, psychological upsets, a tumour even. You need to have your doctor exclude other possible causes by physical examination and routine X-rays, blood tests and so on. But if nothing is found to account for your symptoms and they keep returning in spite of treatment and reassurance, then you should begin to suspect that you may have an allergy to certain foods or environmental chemicals.

Q What is allergy?

A The word means 'altered reaction' and is more or less synonymous with hypersensitivity and idiosyncrasy.

Doctors are divided over allergy; one group (the reductionists) insisting that there must be a demonstrable immunological mechanism underlying the altered response, e.g. antibodies formed against the antigen or allergen.

The others (the clinical ecologists) saying it is enough to identify the offending substance to which the victim is reacting and to show that by avoiding it, symptoms can be averted or reduced.

Q The clinical ecologists seem to take a broader view, but how do they find out what the victim should avoid?

A There are two kinds of allergy; immediate and delayed or cyclical. The immediate variety is obvious to the victim because it is usually something encountered infrequently such as crab-meat, strawberry or a seasonal pollen. Knowing about the allergy from past experience, makes avoidance (or specific desensitization) possible.

Delayed, cyclical allergy occurs when unsuspected sensitivity has developed to something eaten or inhaled day after day, in which case symptoms will be variable and depend on size and timing of dose, and stage of adaptation in which the victim finds himself. In this type of allergy, which is *far* more common, the allergy manifests first as addiction to the very thing which is doing harm. A person in this stage of mal-adaptation to chocolate or milk for example, will get a brief pick-up or relief of tension and other symptoms on eating or drinking the allergen and only feel bad some hours later if another dose of chocolate or milk is not taken.

A further dose will turn off or mask the symptoms, so the victim gets into a cycle of pick-up and hangover just like the alcoholic who is, of course, a good example of a chemical victim hooked on what for him is a self-administered allergen, poisonous in large doses.

The diagnosis of masked allergy is confirmed by abstaining from the chemical or food until symptoms subside – from five to seven days – and then challenging with a dose of the avoided food or drink and observing the result. If the old symptoms return within thirty minutes or so, the allergen has been identified and avoidance of it thereafter will keep symptoms associated with that particular food or chemical away.

This procedure can be followed for a whole range of foods, drinks and chemicals. It is repeatable, objective and convincing, particularly to the patient. The same food will produce different symptoms in different people and different foods will produce different symptoms in the same person – evidence of biochemical individuality.

The phenomenon has been called specific mal-adaptation.

Q   So it is possible to be allergic to common foods or domestic chemicals and not know it until this special avoidance and challenge procedure has been gone through?

A   Yes. The phenomenon of masking explains why. It converts intermittent chronic symptoms to immediate ones of obvious cause, and can be taught to any intelligent chemical victim and used on a do-it-yourself basis provided the symptoms are not too severe.

With disabling symptoms such as asthma, epilepsy and suicidal depression (which would be dangerous if 'turned on' acutely) the testing must be done under medical supervision with nursing help and antidotes at hand.

Q So what should an ordinary member of the public do if he thinks he has a masked allergy?

A First of all, go and talk it over with your family doctor and have him exclude other causes using traditional methods. This is important because common things commonly afflict us and although allergy is very widespread, so is infection. Your cough could be due to a patch of pnuemonia. Scabies or ringworm could account for your chronic skin rash. Then if your doctor has not been able to establish a cause for your complaint, even with the help of hospital specialists, you should raise the question of environmental causes. Ask him 'could it be due to allergy?' His response to this question is crucial. If he dismisses the idea out of hand you are not going to get much help from him. If he will consider the possibility he may be willing to help you do an ecological investigation or refer you to a clinical ecologist who can.

Q I don't want to put his back up. What do I do if he blows his top?

A Try to see his point of view and withdraw gracefully. You need to get away and think, without antagonizing him. He may be one of those GPs who hates what he considers cranky or does not understand, but is a wizard at getting you into hospital quickly if you have something with which he is familiar, like acute appendicitis or a fracture.

Q I like my GP but he is conventional and does not enjoy being told what to do. So can I do it on my own?

A Yes, you can, but you should get your GP's blessing or at least put him in the picture, so that if you run into difficulties and have to call him out, he will know what you have been up to. Then, if possible, you should contact a local branch of Action Against Allergy (see appendix J), read the literature they recommend and if possible get the name and address of a more experienced fellow sufferer who could give you some guidance.

Q What about doctors? Are there any who specialize in this work and can be consulted privately? I do have some private health insurance.

A   Yes there are, and the numbers are growing. At the moment Private Patients Plan will sometimes pay for you to see either a GP or a hospital specialist who practises clinical ecology. BUPA (British United Provident Association) will only pay if the clinical ecologist is a consultant, but they have some claims under review and may eventually pay for you to see a GP ecologist privately. AAA can give you names of suitable doctors.

Q   Supposing I am lucky and find an ecology-minded doctor nearby, will I have to go into a hospital or nursing home to have the tests done?

A   Not necessarily. It depends how bad your symptoms are. I do a lot of this work on an outpatient basis and so do ninety per cent of the clinical ecologists in the USA. Patients with migraine, skin rashes, digestive trouble and things that are not too disabling need not come into hospital. But for ulcerative colitis, severe asthma and some of the more serious psychiatric problems, patients need a hospital bed.

Q   Do you do it on the NHS?

A   Yes – mostly. But I am restricted to patients living within the catchment area of my hospital.

Q   Will you explain how you deal with a case, so that I can see what is involved?

A   OK. First I go through routine questioning designed to get some basic information:

  1   Exactly what symptoms are complained of?

  2   What sort of person is the illness happening to? This means a full biography, during the telling of which a lot of useful information comes out.

  3   Do the symptoms and the history match up with what I know of ecological illness?

  4   Are there any signs of the seven other possible causes of ill health?

      1   congenital (born with it)
      2   traumatic (injury)
      3   degenerative (wearing out)
      4   infective (contagious)
      5   neoplastic (cancer)

6 toxic (poisoning)

7 psychological (psychosomatic)

To rule out these other causes, a general medical history must be taken, a full physical examination carried out and routine special investigations arranged: chest X-ray, haematology (blood count) biochemistry (blood minerals and electrolytes, screening test for VD) etc., but by the time a patient gets to my clinic all these things have usually been done several times over and a label such as 'hysteria', 'functional' or 'psychosomatic' attached. I would like to see patients earlier.

Other specialized colleagues can be consulted at this stage of the routine investigation. The dental surgeon perhaps, if an impacted wisdom tooth is suspected; the radiologist for doubtful X-rays etc. Having satisfied myself that the case probably is ecological (allergic or environmentally triggered) a decision has to be made as to whether to treat the case as an out-patient or in-patient. Five years ago, when the NHS was less short of money and beds were easier to find, I used to admit quite a lot of patients. Now, unless they are very ill indeed, all are treated as out-patients.

Q What difference does it make?

A For one thing, I can spend much more time with an in-patient. The dietician can organize the food and nurses, a junior doctor and medical student can be involved, which makes the whole exercise more interesting. On the other hand, with an out-patient, the relatives and the patient have to take on a lot of responsibility from the beginning, which is probably a good thing, since they are going to have to manage on their own eventually and it is better not to let them get used to having everything organized for them. So necessity has forced me to simplify things and make use of diet sheets and self-scoring charts which can be filled in at home and brought along to the clinic at each appointment.

Q So at what stage do you see the relatives?

A As early as possible. I like to have the spouse and anyone else living in the house (e.g. a grown-up daughter or a sister) come to the first assessment interview to confirm and amplify the story the patient gives. A good clear history is absolutely

essential and some patients are already confused and groggy
when first seen.

Q It sounds time-consuming. Is that difficult?

A I do take longer than average with each new patient. But
it is time well spent if I get the diagnosis right and the regimen
which I prescribe can be followed effectively at home. Once set
on the right course, a patient only has to see me occasionally and
briefly, unless things come badly unstuck. I can see three new
patients in a morning.

Q So you have obtained a full history. What do you do next?

A Find out exactly what goes into the patient's mouth from
the moment of waking to the moment of going to sleep at night.
I am looking especially for repetitive and addictive patterns of
eating, indicative of the beginning of mal-adaptation to food
allergens. Some patients are very poor witnesses and a husband
or wife is needed to sit in and check the accuracy of this vital
dietary information.

GPs and junior hospital doctors will often overlook the most
glaring examples of addictive eating and drinking because they
have not been taught its importance.

One patient who was drinking forty cups of coffee a day said
she drank 'occasional' cups of coffee and another, who never
even mentioned it in his diet history, was found to be consuming
between four and five pounds of salted peanuts a week, mainly
during the evenings in front of the television. Another got
through a whole bottle of Worcestershire sauce every ten days.

Heavy drinkers are notorious for making misleading statements
about their consumption of intoxicants. So much so that those
masters of understatement, the Irish, commonly invite you to take
part in a night-long drinking session by asking you to have 'just
the one'.

Having got an accurate idea of the dietary habits, I then either
fast the patients for five days or put them on a diet which excludes all their addictants, which I call a Stone Age diet (see
appendix C).

*Q With all this addiction to food and drink, how do you persuade
patients to stick to an exclusion diet?*

A It is not easy. The more disabled the patient, the more likely they are to co-operate. But some who are really quite ill would rather put up with their symptoms than give up their addiction.

Q What do you do about people on drugs prescribed by other doctors?

A I try to taper them off during the early part of my treatment. But when a patient has been on regular repeat prescriptions for potent tranquillizers and antidepressants for years, this may cause withdrawal symptoms involving delirium or convulsions. So I may let them continue on a lower dose for some while until they themselves feel the drugs to be no longer necessary.

I try to spot the poorly motivated, screwed-up personalities who will never apply an ecological programme properly. One has to be realistic. It is no good prescribing an exclusion diet and a chemical clean-up of the home and habits if the patient is too clueless or weak-willed to follow instructions faithfully.

It is a question of quality of the underlying intellect and personality, which have more to do with genetics, upbringing and education than with allergy.

I have learned, from bitter experience, that some patients have to be weeded out at the first interview in favour of those with 'better' personalities, more likely to benefit from treatment, because they can be trusted to tell the truth and follow a programme honestly.

Q How do smoking and indoor air pollution with chemicals fit in?

A The chemical side of clinical ecology is even more important than the biological (pollens, moulds, and natural foods). No clinical ecolgogist likes treating a patient who will not stop smoking. It is addictive and causes chemical allergy.

Chemical allergy can occur with prescribed drugs and to things in the indoor atmosphere at home or at work; is penetrating increasingly into food, with the more and more widespread use of chemical additives; and also into our physical environment through the use of sprays, polishes, natural gas and oil for cooking and central heating, etc. I note details of type of house, heating, cooking and ventilating arrangements, situation of boiler, type of motor car and garage (old or new car, separate or integral garage). Use of aerosols, paints, odorous plastics, insect abatement sprays, etc. The idea is to estimate the size of the chemical load to which the patient is having to adapt. Then, before starting the five-day fast or Stone Age exclusion diet, I give them an instruction sheet on how to clean-up their home chemically (see appendix B).

As far as treatment goes, with my limited facilities at the hospital, I have to be content with a sixty to seventy-five per cent cut back in symptoms at best, before carrying out challenges. I am manipulating the stages of adaptation. I take them out of stages two and three (adaptation and early exhaustion) in their battle to adapt to allergenic foods and chemicals by removing as many as possible of their suspect foods, food additives and air-borne chemicals. This puts them back into non-adapted stage one, where they are acutely sensitive to challenge with the avoided substances.

Chronic symptoms have been reduced and the patient made ready to produce acute ones on challenge, for diagnostic purposes. Before doing it, I show them the diagram of the stages of adaptation and a drawing of Bill Rea's barrel effect (see page 152). It is almost self-explanatory: the barrel represents the patient. Symptoms only come on when the level of water overflows. The level can be reduced by turning off the taps or by raising the walls of the barrel (increasing the patient's resistance).

Q All this sounds pretty complicated. Can you simplify it down for home use with some supervision from the GP?

A Yes. With no medical intervention at all, anyone can take the following steps towards better health. Tackle the foods first and then the chemicals.

1 Write down exactly what goes into your mouth on an average day. You will be surprised how repetitive and limited your eating and drinking pattern really is.

2 Cut out all those foods and drinks which you crave and feel you cannot do without. This means going on a Stone Age-type diet (see appendix C).

3 Follow the exclusion diet, keeping a record of your food intake and level of symptoms on the score sheets (appendix C) for one week. You may feel better, after you have got over some withdrawal symptoms during the first two or three days.

4 If you are not much improved, carry out a thorough chemical clean-up of your home (see appendix B). Better still, go away, still following your Stone Age diet, and keeping score sheets, and stay for ten days in a chemically clean area: an all-electric non-polluted house up a hill by the seaside or in some remote country area, to see if you get well. If you do, you will find that on returning home you get worse again. This means your home or workplace is at fault and you must create an especially clean oasis in one room to which you can retire when symptoms get on top of you.

5 To expand your diet and identify your particular food culprits, start challenging yourself with single foods three days apart in the morning before you eat or drink anything else but water and note your reaction on the score sheets which you must continue to fill up daily and file in a folder. A pattern will emerge and you will get to know what to expect from a test feeding with a challenge food. Add the ones that cause no reaction to your list of compatible foods and put the ones to which you react on your banned list.

6 Try to rotate all safe foods through a four-day cycle in order to maintain your tolerance for them.

7 To identify specific chemical allergies, carry out sniff tests (appendix F) on suspect chemicals to which you have been habitually exposed. Foods are grouped in families and you may be allergic to more than one food within a family (see appendix E).

8 If you get an acute reaction to a food or chemical challenge, try to turn it off with a dose of alkaline salts (see appendix G). The sooner you take these the better they work.

Q   This is quite a tough programme. What do I do if I find I just can't avoid some things, or have so many suspect foods that I cannot get enough to eat?

A   You must find an interested doctor and ask him to show you how to de-sensitize yourself. Several doctors in the UK already have the equipment for doing this and as the method becomes

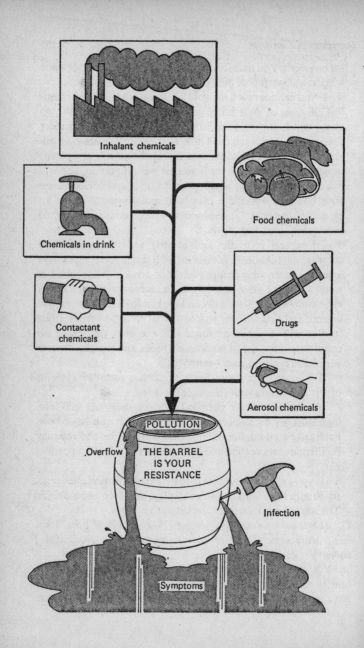

Stages of adaptation to specific substances

1 ALARM (Infrequent Feeding)	2 RESISTANCE (Regular Frequent Feeding)		3 EXHAUSTION (Food may be given up temporarily)
Pre-adaptive, non-adapted and immediately susceptible	*Addicted* 2a *Adapted and tolerant*	2b *Maladapted and becoming intolerant*	*Post-adaptive or non-adapted – very intolerant*
Showing symptoms at once on eating or inhaling the food or chemical, so patient aware of the allergy.	Picked up and pleasantly stimulated on eating or inhaling the addicting substance. Patient unaware of allergy.	Unpleasantly stimulated and rapidly hungover unless increasing doses of the addictant are taken at shorter and shorter intervals.	Each dose followed by immediate onset of symptoms. This stage rarely entered in food allergy, but can be reached in severe chemical allergy and in alcoholism.

Same stages as seen in the ecology clinic

Patient returned to this stage for purpose of challenge after 5 days avoidance of the addictant.	Regarded as normal by patient, friends, colleagues and GP.	All is not well, friends, relatives, patient and GP see this stage as onset of illness.	Patient obviously unwell. Pathological changes may render illness irreversible, with symptoms all the time unless food is given up.

Illness is reversible in Stage 2.
Symptoms intermittent becoming
more frequent in 2b as exhaustion
approaches.

more widely known, more and more allergists and GPs will be able to do it.

Q Are there any other ways of strengthening resistance to food and chemical allergy – ways more accessible to the average person?

A Yes. There are several.

1 Your GP can prescribe Nalcrom (sodium cromoglycate) for you to take before meals to block off the bad effect of allergens in your food. I find that 300 mg (three x 100 mg capsules) fifteen to twenty minutes before food and drink will protect many patients but by no means all. Some react badly to Nalcrom itself or to the gelatine capsule in which it is contained. To avoid this, you can pull the capsule apart and dissolve the cromoglycate powder in water, then drink it. Because so much absorption of food and drink takes place from the mouth, I advise patients to swallow two of the capsules and put the third under the tongue to dissolve slowly and block off receptors in the mouth. Nalcrom solution should be rinsed round the mouth slowly before swallowing to achieve the same result. If your symptoms are also due to inhalant allergy you will need Intal and nasal spray as well.

2 Challenges can be performed with drops of food solutions placed under the tongue for two minutes. This is an alternative to provocation and neutralization of symptoms by the Joe Miller injection technique. It is described in detail in a *Nursing Times* article I wrote with Sue Todd (see page 82).

3 Sublingual challenge and neutralization does not require sterile food extracts and uses real foods, freshly dissolved in distilled water, so a doctor is not required to do them.

A reaction to a sublingual challenge is good evidence of allergy to the food used. No reaction does not always mean that the food is safe when eaten and swallowed. You still have to try it out as a food at a meal to be quite sure that when it gets inside you it does not cause trouble by becoming allergenic during digestion, by reaction with another food, or by forming an upsetting metabolite during or after absorption from the gut.

4 Orthomolecular treatment can help restore enzyme systems to proper working order and thus raise your resistance to food and chemical allergy.

The word 'orthomolecular' means giving large doses of vitamins and minerals already present in the body and essential to its proper working. It is the opposite of the toximolecular treatment used by most doctors when they prescribe lethal drugs in sub-lethal doses to try to stimulate or suppress isolated bits of your biochemistry.

5 Acupuncture. This is an ancient method of healing originating in China thousands of years ago and recently gaining recognition by doctors in the West. I have referred several patients with difficult allergy problems to a medically qualified acupuncturist for strengthening of their resistance and reduction of their level of symptoms. It has helped in some cases. One of the most promising uses of acupuncture in clinical ecology is for turning off the craving for allergenic foods. It works for this and even for heroin addiction in some cases.

6 Hypnosis. Hypnotic suggestion can help reduce cravings and make symptoms more tolerable by inducing relaxation. Dr David Collison, President of the Australian Society of Medical Hypnotherapists, is an authority on this and has started an ecology clinic in Sydney.

7 Other ways of helping chemical victims include osteopathy, homeopathy, natural therapy, faith healing, meditation, relaxation therapy and biofeedback. All have a limited place in treatment but are too complicated to enlarge on here. Practitioners in all these specialities are to be found in Britain and America. My advice about them is that those with recognized medical qualifications are preferable to those without.

Epilogue

'The body is a cell state in which every cell is a citizen. Disease is merely a conflict of the citizens of the state brought about by the action of external forces.'

Rudolph Virchow in *Cellular Pathology* (1858)

Clinical ecology has passed beyond the stage at which it can still be regarded as a fringe subject. It has gained medical respectability in the last few years and many doctors now see its potential. Since the *Lancet* gave it its blessing in a leading article,[27] it has come in from the cold.

Sir Almroth Wright, founder with Sir Alexander Fleming, of the world famous Wright-Fleming Institute at St Mary's Hospital, Paddington in London, once said that a new idea in medicine has to pass through three stages:

1 When it is regarded as ridiculous.
2 When doctors say 'ok it is possible, but where is the proof?'
3 When everyone dismisses it as obvious.

Ted Randolph, in his Herculean struggle to get clinical ecology off the ground in America, has gone through stages one and two during the past forty years and is now slightly bewildered to find that his ideas are at last being accepted.

The Society for Clinical Ecology was strong enough to mount its first international meeting in London at the Royal College of Physicians from 30 May to 1 June 1979. Among the speakers were Professor Jack Pepys, William A. Hemmings, Professor Cedric Wilson, Théron G. Randolph, Gaston Pawan, Ronald Finn, Professor William Rea, and the author.*

*Professor Pepys (p 25) Dr Randolph (p 6) and Professor Rea (p 3) have been introduced earlier in the book. Dr Hemming is head of the Agricultural Research Council Immunology Group, University College

Expert evidence from clinical ecologists has been called in defence of chemical victims who commit crimes while mentally disturbed as a result of cerebral allergy.

On Wednesday 8 March 1978, a young boy was arrested for the attempted murder of his fourteen-year-old sister, who had been stabbed in the back while she lay asleep in bed at her home in a town in mid-western America. The lawyer defending the boy has become an expert on medico-legal aspects of clinical ecology and the role of food and chemical allergens in inducing mental illness and criminal behaviour, and has published an article on the subject for lawyers.[59] The juvenile court permitted Carl's mother (Carl is not his real name) to seek ecological and ortho-molecular treatment for him as an alternative to indefinite incarceration. This treatment was given by Dr Théron Randolph who was one of the attending physicians in the case. She made a film of Carl's progress under treatment and sent me a report about him in June 1979, which she has kindly allowed me to abbreviate and quote:

'He had been depressed constantly, was frequently hostile and had been diagnosed as having schizophrenia with autistic features. He was obese, had a pasty white skin, severe dandruff and oily hair. Dr Randolph found that a whole range of symptoms could be induced by the consumption of specific foods, including tomatoes and bananas. Airborne chemicals and certain waters were shown to be offenders and to contribute to Carl's schizophrenia. By the time his treatment finished, he had become much more socially outgoing and would visit patients in other rooms, introducing himself in a friendly way. He was given an exclusion programme for rehabilitation, to be supervised by his parents at their holiday farm in West Virginia, and at the time of writing has remained well under the course of treatment prescribed.'

of North Wales. Dr Cedric Wilson is Professor of Pharmacology, Trinity College, Dublin. Dr Pawan is Pathologist at the Middlesex Hospital, London, and Dr Finn is Instructor in Medicine at Liverpool University and Consultant Physician to the Royal Liverpool Hospital.

This case was mentioned in the discussion which ended a *Man Alive* television documentary on clinical ecology networked throughout the UK on BBC2 in September 1979. Professor Pepys and I appeared on the programme with other doctors.

Reviewing this programme next day, Herbert Kretzmer, television critic of the *Daily Mail*, wrote, 'If pork, shellfish and cats' hair can provoke extreme physical reactions in allergic sufferers, might not some forms of depression or schizophrenia be susceptible to the same kind of explanation? If found to be true it would put a lot of psychoanalysts out to grass.'

Louise Panton, who produced the programme, told me later that six and a half million people had watched it – a better than average figure for *Man Alive* and good evidence of public interest in the subject.

The saying of Albert Einstein's, about theories being more promising the more widely they can be applied, is apt because the theory of specific adaptation which underlies the practice of clinical ecology is so widely applicable. As my literary agent, Peter Grose of Curtis Brown, said to me: 'Once you know about it, you see it everywhere'; which is true. It explains why migraine sufferers often get a headache if they miss a meal; why alcoholics eventually lose their tolerance and are made ill by drink instead of getting a temporary lift from it; why business men tend to go to sleep after lunch and wake feeling aggressive; why many people who go on holidays to countries with clean air and unchemicalized food feel poorly for two or three days (withdrawal symptoms, not necessarily food poisoning) and then feel incredibly well and can eat everything with relish; why some women feel itchy and uncomfortable in nylon dresses; why weed control lawn sprays may make your muscles ache and feel tired – chemical allergy may well be the answer.

This list could go on and on: hooliganism, shoplifting and road traffic accidents may be triggered by allergy to food, drink and chemical fumes affecting the brain. This is *not* an excuse for wrong-doers; allergy must be objectively and specifically diagnosed in every suspected case.

The theory of clinical ecology is that most human illness is a result of breakdown of inter-related parts of the body due to inability to remain normal in the face of daily exposure to specific chemicals put into our food and drink and into the air we breathe.

Under modern conditions of chemical pollution in the industrialized world the theory continues; our powers of adaptation designed for stone-age conditions are running out. The more susceptible among us are becoming chronically sick.

If this theory is right, then taking the load of environmental chemicals off susceptible, ill people should restore them to health. Putting the chemical load back on, experimentally, should make them ill again. This book describes how it has been done.

The benefits which come from applying the theory of specific adaptation are equalled only by those which came from the germ theory of disease:

● Sense can be made of incomprehensible medical histories.

● The cause of mysterious polysymptomatic syndromes can be established.

● Chronic ill-health of obscure origin can be changed by ecological manoeuvres, to acute illness with demonstrable causes in the physical environment.

● Effective medical treatment with the minimum of drugs is made possible.

● Millions of chronically sick people can be restored to health.

● The worst fears of the ecologists about the hazards of pollution of food, air and water can be confirmed and given medical backing so that political decisions about cleaning up the environment can be taken and implemented.

● The artificial gap between mental and physical illness created by Freud and his followers can be bridged.

● Worthwhile clues to the origins of the modern epidemics of obesity, high blood pressure, coronary thrombosis, rheumatism, digestive disorders, depression and disturbed and violent behaviour can be provided.

● Lines of demarcation between medical specialities can be crossed.

● Clinical research and practice is given a new impetus and direction.

● Prevention and early recognition of disease is possible.

Having demonstrated the cause-and-effect relationship between patients and their chemical environment, clinical ecologists proceed to cure illness by showing how the offending chemicals can be avoided or, if they cannot, how powers of specific adaptation or resistance may be strengthened by immunizing techniques and vitamin/mineral replacement therapy (orthomolecular treatment). Already, some very sick people are being rescued in this way, and the time has come to make clinical ecology more widely available.

This book has described how all this was discovered and how it is put into practice. Polysymptomatic syndromes due to breakdown of specific adaptation have been described and catalogued for all to recognize. If you have a food or chemical allergy problem, I hope this book will help to teach you how to eat, drink, live, breathe and work with less hazard to health. If it contributes to a wider understanding of the value of clinical ecology, I shall be content.

Appendices

These appendices are not intended to give a complete do-it-yourself guide for chemical victims wishing to undertake self-treatment.

In the first place, victims must consult an ecologically oriented doctor to make sure that they really have got ecological illnesses.

There are several good books on self-help for chemical victims, mostly published in the USA, and I have included most of them within the body of the text of this book. The name and publisher of the relevant books is given in the list of references, and AAA will be glad to supply copies and further information. For your convenience a basic reading list is given here:

Human Ecology and Susceptibility to the Chemical Environment, T. G. Randolph MD, Charles C. Thomas, Springfield, Illinois, 1962: essential reading on chemical allergy; hardback.

    Coping with your Allergies, Natalia Golos and Frances Golos Golbitz, Simon & Schuster, New York, 1979: foreword by Dr Randolph; this is a good, practical guide for the non-medical reader; hardback.

    Allergies and the Hyperactive Child, Doris J. Rapp MD, Sovereign Books, New York, 1979: this is a wide-ranging book by a paediatrician aimed at parents and the general reader; hardback.

    Clinical Allergy, Harris Hosen MD, Exposition Press, Hicksville, New York, 1978: aimed more at doctors and nurses. Includes a lot on allergy to dusts and inhalant allergens; hardback.

    Not all in the Mind, Richard Mackarness, Pan Books, 1976: slanted towards psychiatric illness; paperback.

Symptoms of chemical allergy

Here are the criteria for spotting food and chemical allergy. See how many, if any, of your own symptoms fit in.

1 Illness fluctuates

2 Five symptoms that come and go:

  (*a*) Swelling of different parts of the body
  (*b*) Heavy sweating, unrelated to exercise
  (*c*) Fatigue, not helped by rest
  (*d*) Bouts of racing pulse
  (*e*) Marked fluctuations in weight

3 Evidence of food addiction (craving) and repetitive menus

4 Other obvious conventional allergies, e.g. hay fever, urticaria, rashes, headache (often morning), asthma and/or a history of allergy in your family

5 Various food-allergic symptoms referred to particular parts of the body:

Head
Aphthous ulcers in mouth
Halitosis (bad breath)
Nasal catarrh and frequent throat-clearing
Headache – including migraine
Giddiness – including Ménière's disease

Chest
Asthmatic wheezing
Fleeting pains in the breasts, with or without 'mastitis'

Cardio-vascular
Tachycardia (racing pulse)
Arrhythmias (certain types)
Vasculitis (spontaneous bruising or clotting)

Abdominal/digestive
Bloating and discomfort after food
Peptic-ulcer-type pain
Regional ileitis (inflammation of the small intestine)
Bowel cramps and colic
Irritable colon syndrome
Ulcerative colitis
Alternating diarrhoea and constipation
Piles (haemorrhoids)

Genito-urinary
Frequency of urination
'Cystitis' without evidence of infection
Menstrual disorders
Impotence
Frigidity

Musculo-skeletal
'Fibrositis' (aching muscles)
Arthralgia (painful joints)
Backache
'Rheumatism'

Skin
Urticaria (wheels or hives)
Itchy rashes that come and go
Itching and blushing without rash
Oedema (swelling)

Mental
Panic attacks and chronic anxiety
Depression
Hypomania (persistent elation unrelated to circumstances)
Hyperkinesis (overactivity)
Purposeless violence, including 'smashing up'
Nervous tension and mental confusion
Thought disorder (delusions and hallucinations)
Alcoholism

It is not suggested that this list is complete or that any or all of the above conditions are solely caused by food and/or chemical allergy. Hence the insistence on conventional medical examination and investigation before the methods of clinical ecology are applied.

The chemically clean home

People with allergic tendencies should clean up their chemical environment as much as possible. Below are some suggestions to make you aware of the many chemical exposures you come into contact with daily.

Cooking
Use glass, porcelain, enamel ware, iron or stainless steel cookware. Do NOT use teflon, chemically treated utensils or aluminium.

Clothing
Choose natural fibres. Cotton, wool or silk are the best. Avoid nylon, polyesters and other man-made or synthetic materials. Try to use the natural fibres when choosing other fabric items, such as upholstery or floor coverings.

Bedding
Many modern mattresses are treated with moth proofing and conditioning chemicals. It is wise to protect yourself against inhaling these chemicals by covering the mattress with a layer of aluminium foil (shiny side up) and at least four cotton mattress covers. The covers help eliminate exposure to dust and mould too. Choose cotton sheets and blankets. Use pillows filled with cotton flock or discarded cotton garments, shredded. DO NOT ALLOW ANY FOAM RUBBER ARTICLES ON THE BED ON WHICH YOU ARE SLEEPING! Remove from your bedroom any items which contain any form of synthetics, such as foam backed hangings, foam backed rugs or cushions.

Floor covering
Wood, lineoleum and ceramic tiles or terrazzo are the best choices. Fitted carpeting holds dust whereas cotton scatter rugs

can be shaken out regularly. Choose wool or cotton carpeting over other fibres.

Pest control
There is no entirely satisfactory method at this time. Try to avoid petrochemicals, such as used in 'killer sprays, if it is at all possible. Pyrethrum is the safest, in a water-based mist.

Painting
Latex paint is the best choice. Mix 500 g of baking soda with 5 litres of paint before applying it. Try to avoid being exposed to new paint until the fumes have had time to 'gas out'.

Heating
Electric is the best choice or hot water pipes. If you are installing a new system, be sure there is no glued-in insulation which would cause fumes. A good filter system is strongly recommended. Gas heating should be avoided. Site the boiler (however it is fired) in an outhouse away from your living quarters.

Water
Use water from a deep well, or uncontaminated source. Make sure no chemicals are added to your drinking water. Use spring water bottled in glass, or distilled. If drinking distilled water all the time, take a pinch of sea salt daily to guard against mineral deficiency.

APPENDIX C

The Stone Age diet

Follow this diet strictly for one week recording everything you eat or drink from the moment you wake to when you go to sleep at night (a chart is given on page 170).

Breakfast
Fresh apple, pears, banana or orange or grapefruit. Fructose if liked to sweeten. Grilled fish, e.g. plaice, cod, hake or trout cooked in olive oil with lemon – or grilled chops, steak or kidneys. Fried tomatoes, mushrooms or potatoes. Spring water or herbal tea to drink.

Mid-morning
Fresh fruit.
Herb tea or spring water.

Lunch
Roast beef, lamb or pork, or grilled steak or chops or fresh game, or grilled or fried fish using olive oil, or grilled or fried liver or kidney.
Good serving fresh green vegetable, e.g. cabbage, sprouts, cauliflower, broccoli, spinach.
Root vegetables: e.g. carrot, swedes, turnip or parsnip.
Potatoes plain boiled or cooked in jackets or mashed, with olive oil, salt and fresh ground pepper or fried in olive oil.
Fresh fruit.

Supper
Choice of meat or fish as luncheon.
Salad or serving of cooked vegetables.
Serving of potato.
Fresh fruit as liked.
Fresh nuts (in the shell).

Chicory or dandelion coffee (without lactose) or herbal tea.
Malvern or other bottled spring water.

ALLOWED

Fresh meat
Lamb, beef, pork, turkey, goose, duck, pheasant, pigeon,
partridge, venison, rabbit, hare, free range fresh chicken, liver,
kidney, heart.

Fresh fish
All kinds.

Fresh vegetables
Including potato.

All fresh fruit
Preferably home grown or from a farm where sprays are not
used. Commercial fruit must be washed and if heavily contaminated, peeled before eating.

Drinks
Preferably bottled spring water, e.g. Perrier or Schweppes
Malvern Water. Tap water should be boiled or filtered. Herb
teabags, camomile, linden flower, peppermint etc. can be used.
Dandelion coffee (without lactose and not instant).

Seasoning
Fresh ground pepper. Sea salt.

Olive oil
For cooking and salad dressing with lemon juice.

Fructose (for sweetening)

Fresh nuts

FORBIDDEN

Anything manufactured, processed, sprayed, added to or adulterated chemically.

Cereals – wheat, barley, oats, rice, millet, corn, corn oil, biscuits, bread, cakes.

Sugar, sweets, chocolate, fizzy drinks, fruit squashes.

Milk cream, butter, margarine, eggs, cheese.

Canned meat or fish.

Bacon, kippers, smoked fish.

Crisps, packaged nuts.

Coffee, tea, alcohol.

When clear of symptoms on this diet, single items from the forbidden list may be added to the menu, on a test basis, three days apart. If no reaction occurs within three hours the food may be assumed safe and can be eaten in rotation with other safe foods.

LIST ALL FOODS, DRINKS AND MEDICATIONS, NOTE TIMES IN APPROPRIATE COLUMNS, FILL IN SYMPTOMS
AND SCORE SYMPTOMS 0 - 3. (0 = NONE, 1 = SLIGHT, 2 = MODERATE, 3 = SEVERE)

	TIME	FOODS AND DRINKS	UNUSUAL STRESS-CAUSING OCCURRENCES	MEDICINES											
ON WAKING															
BEFORE BREAKFAST															
BREAKFAST															
BETWEEN BREAKFAST AND LUNCH															
LUNCH															
BETWEEN LUNCH AND TEA															
TEA															
BETWEEN TEA AND SUPPER															
SUPPER															
BETWEEN SUPPER AND BEDTIME															
DURING THE NIGHT IF WAKEFUL															

PATIENT'S NAME.................... DATE..................

BASINGSTOKE DISTRICT HOSPITAL
CLINICAL ECOLOGY
RESEARCH UNIT.

Rotary diet

This diet is designed to ensure that you do not eat the same foods and their additives and contaminants day after day thus avoiding a build-up of potentially allergenic substances in the intestines to the point where your tolerance might break down and you would have symptoms. Ideally, no food should be eaten more than once in four days.

Each line represents a single food family (see appendix E). Try not to take more than four different foods at any one meal, but eat as much as you want of each food as its turn comes up. Sea salt can be taken every day and used in cooking. Do not use a lot of extra salt unless the weather is really hot and you are sweating. Avoid any food to which you know you are allergic.

Days 1, 5, 9 etc.

Fruits	Citrus: lemon, orange, grapefruit
Vegetables	Carrots, parsnips, celery, parsley; beet, spinach, spring greens
Meat	Birds: chicken, turkey, duck, goose and eggs
Spices	Black and white peppercorns; celery seed, dill, fennel, caraway
Nuts	Walnuts, pecans
Sweeteners	Date sugar
Drinks and soups	Comfrey or fennell tea; juices made from any of above fruits and vegetables (without added sweeteners)
Cooking fats	Coconut oil or fat from birds listed

Days 2, 6, 10 etc.

Fruits	Grapes and raisins (without sulphur dioxide); strawberries, raspberries, blackberries, loganberries

Vegetables	Cucumber, marrow, courgette; peas, beans, lentils
Meat	All pork products: pork, ham, bacon (not pre-packed or heavily smoked)
Seafood	Mussels, winkles, scallops, oysters.
Spices	Licquorice; sea salt
Nuts	Cashew, pistachio; hazelnuts, filberts
Sweeteners	Carob syrup
Drinks and soups	Indian tea; juices made from any of above fruits and vegetables (without added sweeteners)
Cooking fats	Soya bean oil or fat from pork

Days 3, 7, 11 etc.

Fruits	Apples, pears, quinces; mulberries, figs; rhubarb; currants (black, red, white); gooseberries
Vegetables	Lettuce, chicory, endive, artichoke; potato, tomato, aubergine, green and red peppers; onion, leek, chives, asparagus
Meat	Lamb, rabbit, hare
Fish	Herring, salmon, trout, mackerel
Sweetener	Honey (pure without added sugar)
Drinks and soups	Mint tea; juices from any of above fruits and vegetables (without added sweeteners)
Cooking fats	Safflower seed oil; sesame seed oil
Miscellaneous	Cheese made from sheep's milk (e.g. Rocquefort)

Days 4, 8, 12 etc.

Fruits	Plums, cherries, peaches, apricots; cranberries; papaya
Vegetables	Turnip, radish, cabbage, broccoli, sprouts;

	avocado pear
Meat	Beef, veal
Spices	Mustard, horseradish
	cinnamon, bay leaf; sea salt
Nuts	Almonds
Grains	Wheat, barley, oats, rye, corn, rice
Sweeteners	Cane sugar, corn syrup, glucose
Drinks and	Lemon verbena tea;
soups	matté tea;
	milk;
	juices from above fruits and vegetables (without added sweetener)
Cooking fat	Butter
Miscellaneous	Cheese made from cows' milk

This way of presenting the rotary diet is borrowed from my friend and colleague Dr Doris Rapp, who uses it in her marvellous book, *Allergies and the Hyperactive Child*. Permission to use it is gratefully acknowledged.

Food families

A person allergic to one food is usually allergic to other foods of the same family. This is especially true of plant foods. Peanuts, for example, belong to the pea or legume family, and people who cannot eat peanuts usually cannot eat beans and peas. But they are not necessarily allergic to other nuts. Patients allergic to wheat are often allergic to rice and barley and other grains, but not to buckwheat, a member of another family. Potatoes are related to tomatoes, but not to sweet potatoes. Almonds are related to peaches, but not to pecans. Tuna and salmon are true fish and are related to each other, but not to clams or crabs. And clams and crabs are not related. Tea and coffee are not related, but chocolate and cola (used in cola drinks) are. Carrots and celery are relatives; black pepper and red pepper are not. These and other relationships are shown in the following list. The more important foods are given in capitals.

PLANT FAMILIES

Apple APPLE, PEAR
Buckwheat BUCKWHEAT, RHUBARB
Cashew CASHEW NUT, PISTACHIO, mango
Citrus ORANGE, LEMON, LIME, GRAPEFRUIT, TANG-
ERINE
Cola Nut CHOCOLATE, COLA
Fungi Yeast, edible fungi (inhalant moulds are related to yeast)
Goosefoot BEET, SPINACH, Swiss chard
Gourd (*Melon*) WATERMELON, CUCUMBER, courgette, pumpkin, squash
Grass (*Grains, Cereals*) WHEAT, CORN, RICE, OATS,

BARLEY, RYE, millet, wild rice, brown cane, sugar, bamboo sprouts, malt

Heath BLUEBERRY, CRANBERRY, sloes

Laurel CINNAMON, BAY LEAF, avocado

Legume PEAS, BLACK-EYED PEAS, NAVY BEANS, LIMA BEANS, STRING BEANS, PEANUTS, licorice

Lily ONION, GARLIC, ASPARAGUS, chives, leek

Mallow Okra

Mint MINT, SAGE, THYME, PEPPERMINT, SPEARMINT, OREGANO, basil, horehound, marjoram, savory rosemary

Mustard MUSTARD, TURNIP, RADISH, HORSERADISH, CABBAGE, CAULIFLOWER, BROCCOLI, BRUSSELS SPROUTS, Chinese cabbage, kale, watercress, kohlrabi

Myrtle ALLSPICE, CLOVE

Nightshade TOMATO, POTATO, GREEN AND RED PEPPER, AUBERGINE, TOBACCO, cayenne, paprika, pimiento, chili (peppercorns are not part of this family)

Palm COCONUT, DATE

Parsley CARROT, CELERY, PARSNIP, PARSLEY, DILL, CELERY, SEED, CUMIN, CORIANDER, caraway, anise, angelica, fennel

Plum ALMOND, PLUM (prune), PEACH, APRICOT, CHERRY, nectarine

Rose STRAWBERRY, BLACKBERRY, RASPBERRY, other bramble berries

Sunflower LETTUCE, chicory, endive, Jerusalem artichoke, dandelion, sunflower seeds, tarragon. Ragweed, and pyrethrum are related inhalants

Walnut BLACK and ENGLISH WALNUT, PECAN

PLANT FOODS WITHOUT RELATIVES

These foods represent the only members of their families that are commonly eaten. They therefore are not related to each other or to other foods on this list:

BANANA, BRAZIL NUT, COFFEE, CURRANTS, FIG,

GINGER, GOOSEBERRY, GRAPE, (RAISINS), HAZEL-
NUT, HONEY, NUTMEG, OLIVE, PEPPERCORNS,
PINEAPPLE, SWEET POTATO, TEA, VANILLA, arrow-
root, capers, chestnut, elderberry, juniper, karaya gum, maple
sugar, papaye, persimmon, poppyseed, saffron, sesame seed,
tapioca, wintergreen.

Chemical testing at home

The 'sniff' or inhalation test is an effective way for you to determine your sensitivity to common chemicals in your environment. You will have many of these chemicals on hand; others you can purchase from a chemist.

Plan to test the following chemicals:
1 chlorine (bleach); 2 phenol (carbolic or Jeyes fluid); 3 formaldehyde; 4 alcohol (ordinary surgical spirit); 5 insecticide (take spray can outdoors before spraying into test jar); 6 your favourite perfume and cigarette smoke (test by asking a friend to smoke a cigarette in your presence).

Purchase at least four small glass jars with lids or stoppers from a pharmacy. Place a small amount of cotton wool in the bottom of each jar. Put five drops of the test chemicals on to each of the cotton wool balls. Seal the jar. Leave the substance sealed up, all prepared, for four days before opening for testing.

Purchase notebook for recording pulses and reactions. Find a clock with a sweep second hand so that the time for each test is accurate.

Select a definite place for all your chemical tests. For good results, use a spot in which there are as few odours as possible. The room should have good ventilation and be away from possible distractions. A backporch or patio area works well. If the sniff causes a reaction, you can then leave the odour and go inside.

Sit in a comfortable chair. Take your pulse by placing the second or third finger of one hand on the artery in your wrist. If you take your pulse at the wrist, slight pressure will help you to count each beat. Count for a full sixty seconds. Faithfully record each pulse five minutes before each test and five, ten, twenty and forty minutes after each test.

Test only one chemical a day. Hold the bottle 30 cm from your nose. Remove the top. Take a sniff. Record your pulse. Take another sniff at five minutes and one last sniff at ten minutes. If you react, stop testing. Record all physical and mental symptoms in your notebook.

It is important that you expose yourself only to the amount of chemical suggested, at the distance recommended, and for the length of time suggested. If you experience any symptoms, stop and record results. Then, begin immediately to clear yourself of the reaction, by exercising in the fresh air.

Several non-toxic remedies will help clear you of symptoms if a reaction to a chemical becomes severe. See appendix G.

Clearing symptoms in an allergic reaction

Three non-toxic remedies will help clear you of symptoms if a reaction to a food occurs:

1 If you have just eaten a food, induce vomiting by sticking your fingers down your throat.

2 Inhale oxygen if you have access to a cylinder, mask and flowmeter, at seven litres per minute, until you feel better. Or take a walk in the fresh air breathing deeply.

3 Take alkali salts: sodium bicarbonate, sodium and potassium bicarbonate, in proportion 2:1 or tri-salts (sodium, potassium and calcium bicarbonate in proportions 2:1:1).

Mix two heaped teaspoons of any of these salts in a full glass of water and drink it, followed by a glass of plain water. This may have a laxative effect and will act as a general antidote. Do not use this treatment more than twice in any one day.

As a laxative to clear the bowel of an offending food, take epsom salts or milk of magnesia in whatever dose you generally use. A warm water enema may also be given, preferably bottled spring or distilled water if that has been used during the test period.

APPENDIX H

Common chemicals in your environment

Chemicals are everywhere in today's environment. Food, water, air, medicines, household cleansers, home furnishings – virtually everything contains chemical additives or synthetic substances.

On the next several pages are listed five of the most common chemicals and the products in which they are found. If you have allergies, it is likely that you are sensitive to some or many of these chemicals.

ALCOHOL

Ethyl alcohol or *ethanol* is formed in wine or cider by fermentation. Industrial ethyl alcohol may be made from molasses, potatoes, grain or organic substances such as shellac and oil. It is used as an ingredient in tinctures and in toilet and drug preparations. It is used in making rubber and ether and used to sterilize surgical instruments. Surgical spirit is methyl alcohol and very poisonous.

Amyl alcohol is made from ethyl alcohol and is used as a solvent.

Isopropyl alcohol is used in the manufacture of anti-freeze, rubbing alcohol and solvents.

Glycerol is found in sweeteners and preservatives in foods. It is used in the manufacture of cosmetics, skin emollients and perfumes; inks, certain glues and cements; many medicines and suppositories.

Menthol is found in perfumes, candies and confections, liquers, and cold medications, where it has a cooling effect on mucous membranes. It is also used in mentholate cigarettes.

CHLORINE

Chlorine is a gas, first made in 1774. It combines readily with many other substances. Uses of chlorine include: water purification, as in drinking water and swimming pools; bleaching; certain textiles for pulp for paper; fire extinguishers; anaesthetics, antiseptics, and disinfectants; cleaning fluids, manufacture of dyes, drugs and cellulose acetate; refining of oil and sugar.

PERFUMES

The composition of a perfume depends upon its usage. Most expensive perfumes contain rare flower oils. Perfumes in soap and in inexpensive perfumes come from man-made materials. There are three basic types of perfumes: extracts or essences (scents), colognes and toilet water. Scents are 10 to 20 per cent perfume dissolved in alcohol. Colognes are 3 to 5 per cent perfume oil dissolved in 80 to 90 per cent alcohol with water making up the balance. Toilet water is 2 per cent perfume oil in 60 to 80 per cent alcohol with the balance in water.

Most perfumes are blends of flower oils, animal substances, synthetics, alcohol and water. Oils from plant substances are extracted by steam distillation. Animal substances are obtained by slow evaporation of substances such as castor from the beaver, civet from the animal of the same name, musk from the male musk deer and ambergris from the sperm whale. Other raw materials may be obtained from natural sources, petrochemicals or coal tar. Alcohol is added to animal or plant substances and then heated. Water is used for dilution.

Products that may contain perfumes include toilet paper, face tissues, lipstick and other cosmetics, body deodorants, room deodorizers and candles.

PHENOL (CARBOLIC)

Phenol is a basic organic chemical and is a constituent of herbicides and pesticides; bakelite moulded articles such as telephones and toys; synthetic detergents; perfumes; petrol, dyes, photography solutions; and preservatives in medications and allergy antigen serum. Phenol is used in the production of epoxy and phenolic resins, aspirin and other drugs and in the manufacture of nylon, polyurethane and explosives.

FORMALDEHYDE

Formaldehyde is found in antiperspirants, dentifrice antiseptic, mouthwashes, germicidal and detergent soaps, hair setting lotions, shampoos and air deodorants. It is used as a disinfectant to destroy bacteria, fungi, moulds and yeasts in the fermentation industry, in the manufacture of antibiotics, in hospital sickrooms and for cleaning surgical instruments.

Formaldehyde improves colour stability of dyed fabrics. It is used in the synthesis of dyes, stripping agents and various chemicals in the dye industry.

Formaldehyde makes natural and synthetic fibres wrinkle-resistant, water-repellant, dye-fast, flame-resistant, shrink-proof, moth-proof and more elastic.

Formaldehyde improves the wet strength and water resistance of paper products. It is used as a preservative and accelerator for photographic developing solutions and as a resin in nail polish.

Formaldehyde is used in the insecticidal solutions for killing flies, mosquitoes and moths and in rodent poisons. It is used in the formulation of slow-release nitrogen fertilizers and as a tanning agent.

Formaldehyde is an additive in concrete, plaster and related products. It is a component part in wallboard, synthetic resins, wood veneer and wood preservatives.

Formaldehyde is used in the synthesis of vitamin A and to improve the activity of vitamin E preparations.

Formaldehyde makes up fifty per cent of the estimated total aldehydes in polluted air. Aldehydes react further to form additional pollutants like smog. The major sources of aldehyde pollution are incomplete combustion of hydrocarbons in petrol and diesel engines and the burning of fuels and incineration of waste. Formaldehyde is the principal agent responsible for burning eyes in smog and in tear gas.

INSECTICIDE

Most pesticides fall into two chemical groups, chlorinated hydrocarbons and organophosphates. The chlorinated hydrocarbons include chlordane, aldrin, dieldrin, endrin, lindane and DDT. The most deadly poisons are derived from organophosphates and include parathion, phosdrin, diazinon and tetraethyl hydrophosphate.

You encounter insecticides in greengrocers, garden shops, orchards and farms, riding stables, warehouses, cinemas, theatres and hotels. Products contaminated with insecticides include tobacco, rubber bands and other rubber products, wool products, packing cases, houseplants and sprayed crops.

Chemical substitutes

Laundry agents For machine-washing clothes, rub damp bicarbonate of soda into dirty spots, then add $\frac{1}{2}$ cup baking soda to one medium washer load of clothes; for particularly dirty clothes, wash with usual washing powder and add $\frac{1}{2}$ cup bicarbonate of soda to rinse cycle, followed by second rinse of clear water. Borax is used with success by some people.

Household cleanser Dampen sink, lavatory or bath. Sprinkle with bicarbonate of soda. Scrub with sponge. For particularly difficult jobs, clean with borax and then baking soda.

Oven cleaner Sprinkle a small amount of water in oven, then sprinkle ample amount of bicarbonate of soda all over. Leave for 30 minutes. Use steel wool pads and small amount of water to loosen dirt. Wipe clean with sponge.

Brass and copper polish Dampen metal object. Apply bicarbonate of soda with sponge. Polish with soft cloth.

Glass and mirror cleaner Dampen cloth with vinegar and wipe off windows.

Fabric softener Fill basin with three parts water to one part vinegar. Allow to soak overnight. Rinse vinegar out of fabric.

Floor polish Choose one that has a higher percentage of the natural wax. Pure beeswax is ideal.

Room deodorizer Partially fill bowls with bicarbonate of soda or vinegar and distribute about room. Potpourri smell nicer and are just as good.

Refrigerator freshener Leave box of bicarbonate of soda open in refrigerator. Change boxes frequently.

Storing or freezing food Store foods in glass or in bags made from the wood fibre cellophane not plastic.

Dishes and cookware Porcelain, glass and stainless steel do not evaporate or transmit chemicals from themselves to the food within.

Carpet pad Use felt under rugs or natural fibre carpet. Rubber or synthetic carpet pad is a major source of evaporation, particularly when heated by sunlight or heat within the house. Carpeting may be made of wool or cotton. Oriental rugs are usually tolerable, especially older, antique rugs.

Deodorant Dip face cloth in a weak solution of bicarbonate of soda and water and apply to underarms.

Toothpaste Mix one part salt with two parts bicarbonate of soda. Apply direct to toothbrush.

Mouthwash Mix one teaspoon bicarbonate of soda with a glass of water. Rinse with tea made from sage or birch leaves.

Toothache Apply oil of cloves directly to tooth.

Hiccups Drink tea made from dill leaves.

Sore throat Mix apple juice and honey. Heat and sip.

Colds, nasal congestion Mix apple juice and honey. Heat and sip.

Earache Heat a teaspoonful of olive oil. Add powdered oregano to the oil. Drop in to ear, close with cotton wool.

Stomach ache, indigestion Mix one teaspoon bicarbonate of soda in glass of water. Drink, then follow with another glass of water. Or drink tea made from camomile or fennel.

Disinfectant Apply garlic juice or a tea made from comfrey or marigold flowers around fresh wounds or cuts.

Sunburn, sprains, frostbite Apply witch hazel liberally.

AAA (ACTION AGAINST ALLERGY),
43 The Downs, London SW20. Tel: 01 947 5082

AAA Book Department through Merton Book Junkantique provides a unique service of information by either supplying directly or giving information as to where the following additive-free materials can be found:

1 Honey (pure). Most commercial honey is made from bees fed on sugar.
2 Coffee substitutes (non instant).
3 Tea substitute (tastes exactly like tea).
4 Cocoa substitute.
5 Bread substitutes (completely gluten-free). Many gluten-free products on the market are not completely gluten-free.
6 Cereal substitutes (completely gluten-free).
7 Roughage (gluten-free).
8 Grains (whole as substitute for breakfast cereals, gluten-free).
9 Flour substitutes (gluten-free).
10 Sprouting seeds (have more enzyme content) can be used as cooked vegetables or salads.
11 Milk substitutes (in powder and paste form and frozen).
12 Meat (additive-free).
13 Salt substitutes
14 Vegetables (organically grown).
15 Air purifyers.
16 Vitamins (additive-free).
17 Minerals (additive-free).
18 Cosmetics (additive-free).
19 Wool (pure).
20 Silk (pure).
21 Cotton (pure).
22 Clothes (non-synthetic).
23 Cotton covers for mattresses.

References

1   Adolph, E. F., 'General and specific characteristics of physiological adaptations', *American Journal of Physiology*, *184*, 1956, pp 18–28

2   Burton, R., *Anatomy of Melancholy*, 1621

3   Brown, E. A., and Colombo, N. J., 'The asthmathogenic effects of odors, smells and fumes', *Annals of Allergy*, *12*, 1954, pp 14–24

4   Blackley, C. H., '*Experimental researches on Catarrhus Aestivus (Hay fever or Hay Asthma)*', Baillière, Tindall and Cox, London, 1873

5   Cleverdon, Mrs S., *Woman's Own* article, 25 June 1977

6   Carroll, Dr M. and Bullock Dr T., 'Rheumatoid and osteoarthritis controlled by ecological management', 12th Advanced Seminar in Clinical Ecology, Miami, 20 November 1978

7   Carson, Rachel, *Silent Spring*, Penguin, 1970

8   *Daily Mail*, letter, 2 February 1979

9   *Daily Telegraph*, 2 March 1979

10 Doerr, R., 'Anaphylaxis, Handbuch der Technik und Methodik der Immunitatslehre', *Forschung*, *2*, 1909, p 856

11 Dohan, F. C., 'Cereals and Schizophrenia', *Acta Psychiatrica Scandinavica*, *42*, 1966, pp 125–152

12 Doll, R. and Hill, B. A., 'Smoking and Carcinoma of the Lung', preliminary report, *British Medical Journal*, 30 September 1950, pp 746–8. Also 'A study of the aetiology of carcinoma of the lung', *British Medical Journal*, 13 December 1952

13 Ellis, N. R., David, R. E. and Denton, C. A., 'The use of antibiotics, hormones, tranquillizers and other chemicals in animal production', Symposium on the nature and fate of chemicals applied to the soil, plants and animal production, USDA Agricultural Research Service, September 1960, p 45

14 Feingold, Ben, 'Recognition of food additives as a cause of symptoms of allergy', *Annals of Allergy*, *26*, 1968, p 309

15 Haeckel, E., *Generelle Morphologie der Organismen*, G. Reimer, Berlin, 1866

16 Hall, Prof Ross Hume, *Food for Nought – the decline of nutrition*, Harper and Row, New York, 1974 (Information for this table was supplied by Maple Leaf Mills Ltd, Toronto, Canada)

17 *Hansard*, 5 May 1979

18 Hansel, W. et al, 'The Isolation and Identification of the Causative Agent in Bovine Hyperkeratosis (X disease) from a processed wheat concentrate'. *Cornell Veterinarian*, *45*, 1955, p 94

19 Huxley, Aldous, *Brave New World*, Penguin, 1960

20 Jenner, E., *An inquiry into the causes and effects of variolae accinae*, 1798

21 Kekwick, A. and Pawan G., 'The Effect of Isocaloric Diets on Weight Loss in the Obese', *The Lancet*, July 1956

22 Kenton, Leslie, 'The Chemistry of Consciousness', *Harpers & Queen*, January 1979

23 Kety, S. S., 'Dietary Factors and Schizophrenia', *Annals of Internal Medicine*, *84*, 1976 p 745

24 Krantz, J. C. Jr and Carr, C. J., *The Pharmacological Principles of Medical Practice*, Williams and Wilkins, 1954

25 *The Lancet*, editorial, 16 August 1969

26 *The Lancet*, *2*, 1976, p 136

27 *The Lancet*, editorial, 3 February 1979

28 Lane, M., 'Did you enjoy your breakfast?', *Sunday Telegraph*, 17 March 1979

29 Lockey, S. D., 'Allergic reactions to F. D. and C. dyes used as colouring and identifying agents in various medications', *Bulletin of Lancaster General Hospital*, Lancaster, Pennsylvania, 1948

30 Lockey, S. D., 'Reactions to hidden agents in foods, beverages and drugs', *Annals of Allergy*, *29*, September 1971, p 461

31 Lockey, S. D., 'Clinical sensitizing properties of food and other commercial products', paper given at the 28th Annual Congress of the American College of Allergists, Dallas, Texas, 9 March 1972, pp 4–5

32 Mackarness, R., 'Stone-Age diet for functional disorders', *Medical World*, *91*, 1959, pp 14–19

33 Mackarness, R., *Eat Fat and Grow Slim*, Harvill Press, London, 1958 and Fontana, 1961 (revised 1976)

34 Mackarness, R., 'The allergic factor in alcoholism', *International Journal of Social Psychiatry*, autumn 1972, p 194

35 Mackarness, R., *Not All in the Mind*, Pan Books Ltd, London, 1976

36 Miller, Joe, *Food Allergy. Provocative Testing and Injection Therapy*, Charles C. Thomas, Springfield, Illinois, 1972

37 Morton Sandler, 'The dopamine hypothesis revisited', from *The Biological Basis of Schizophrenia*, edit. Hemming, W. A., MTP Press Ltd, Lancaster, 1978

38 Noon, L., 'Prophylactic inoculation against hay fever', *The Lancet, 1*, 1911, p 1572

39 Pirquet, C. von., 'Allergie', *Munchener Med. Wochenschrift, 53*, 1906, p 1457

40 Pirquet, C. von and Schick, B., *Die Serumkrankheit*, Leipzig and Vienna, 1905

41 Portier, P. and Richet, C., 'De l'Action Anaphylactique à Certains Venins', *Compt. Rend. Soc. de Biol., 54*, 1902, p 170

42 Randolph, T. G., 'Allergic-type reactions to industrial solvents and liquid fuels; mosquito abatement fogs and mists; motor exhausts; indoor utility gas and oil fumes; chemical additives of food and drugs, and synthetic drugs and cosmetics', *Journal of Laboratory and Clinical Medicine, 44*, 1954, pp 910–14

43 Randolph, T. G., 'Depressions caused by home exposures to gas combustion products of gas, oil and coal', *Journal of Laboratory and Clinical Medicine, 46*, 9 February 1955

44 Randolph, T. G., *Human Ecology and Susceptibility to the Chemical Environment*, Charles C. Thomas, Springfield, Illinois, 1962

45 Rea, W. J., 'Environmentally triggered Cardiac Disease', *Annals of Allergy, 40*, 1978, p 243

46 *Reader's Digest* (Canadian edition), 'You and your heart. 1. The Real Role of Fats', October 1972, pp 59–62

47 Rinkel, H. J., Randolph, T. G. and Zellar, M., *Food Allergy*, Charles C. Thomas, Springfield, Illinois, 1951

48 Roche Lynch, G., *Chemistry and Industry*, 1951, pp 923–33

49 Rowe, A. H., *Food Allergy, its manifestations, diagnosis and treatment, with a general discussion of Bronchial Asthma*, Lea and Febiger, Philadelphia, 1931

50 Schaudin, F. and Hoffman, E., 'Vorlaufiger Bericht uber das Vorkommen von Spirochaeten in Syphilitischen Krankheit-produkten und bei Papillomen', *Arbeit Klinische Gesundheitsamte, 22*, 1905, pp 527–34

51 Selye, H., 'The General Adaptation Syndrome and the Disease of Adaptation', *American Journal of Allergy, 17*, 1946

52 Taylor, G. S. and Hern, W. S., 'Cardiac Arrhythmias due to aerosol propellants', *Journal of the American Medical Association*

53 Todd, S. and Mackarness, R., 'Allergy to Food and Chemicals

Part 1', *Nursing Times*, *16*, 1978, p 438, 'Part 2', *Nursing Times*, *23*, 1978, p 506

54 Tomlin, P. J., 'Health problems of anaesthetists and their families in the West Midlands', *British Medical Journal*, *1*, 3 March 1979, pp 779–84

55 Werch, S. C., letter in *Journal of the American Medical Association*, *187*, 14 March 1964, p 872

56 William, Dr R. J., *Biochemical Individuality*, University of Texas Press, 1956

57 *Worthing Gazette*, 13 December 1978

58 Yevick, P., 'Oil Pollutants in Marine Animals', 8th Advanced Seminar in Clinical Ecology, Instatape 11, 1975

59 Feldman, James K., 'Memorandum to Co-Counsel on Orthomolecular Psychiatry', *Journal of Orthomolec. Psych.*, *5*, *4*, 1978, pp 281–5

Index

abdominal pain 8
acetylcholine 139–40
Action Against Allergy 145, 146, 186
active immunity 35
acupuncture 155
adaptation, to allergens 82, 84–5, 112, 133, 158
 specific adaptation syndrome 85
 stages of 84–6, 150, 153
 to gas and gas-related chemicals 108–9
addiction 24, 124–5, 144, 148
 masking basis of 85
Adolph, Professor E. F. 84
adrenalin, adrenal hormones 36, 41, 42, 84
aerosol sprays 3, 4, 25, 79, 98, 112, 114, 124, 125, 127, 128, 149, 150
aggression, uncontrolled 7
air pollution 81, 98, 159
 indoor 104–14, 123, 149–50
Albert, Prince of Monaco 37
alcohol 108, 175, 178
alcoholism 24, 107, 119, 120, 157, 163
alcohols, in food additives 102
Alexander, Andrew 27
'all-in-the-mind' approach 119
allergens,
 chemicals as 44, 45, 70
 drugs as 37, 42
 in the air 68, 81
 in drinking water 68
 in food 39, 44, 62, 68, 76
 inhalant 39, 62, 81
 neutralization of 52
 responses, individual 50
allergy 37, 38, 41, 43, 60
 anaphylactic allergy 41
 and side-chain theory of immunity 41
 caused by environment 5, 21, 43
 defined 22, 38–9, 143
 'hair of the dog' phenomenon 81–2, 85, 107
 immediate and cyclical allergy 143–4
 masked allergy 24, 97, 144, 145, see also masking
 term introduced 38, 41
 testing for 85, 144, 176–7
 to smells 113–14
 treatment of 145–55
allergy, adaptation to 82, 84–5, 112, 133, 158
 specific adaptation syndrome 85
 stages of 84–6, 150, 153
 to gas and gas-related chemicals 108–9
allergy, chemical 1, 6, 7, 9, 10, 11fn, 12, 15, 24, 42, 43, 70, 112, 140, 149
 adaptation to 84
 and drugs 37, 42, 95

allergy, chemical, *continued*
  side effect of food marketing 66
  symptoms of 162–3
  testing for 78, 79
allergy, food xv, 6, 7, 8–9, 10,
    11fn, 12, 24, 39, 49, 51, 140
  adaptation and 84
  antidotes to 62–3
  as cause of disease 123, 171
  cause of obesity 9, 77
  masked 24, *see also* masking
  testing for 78–9
  treatment of 58–62
allergy, inhalant 39, 62, 81, 112,
    124
allergy, investigation of 3, 14,
    39, 45
  skin tests 9, 39, 47, 49
  two schools 39
Allergy Group 51
amaranth dye 57
amino acids 31
amitryptidine 94
ammonium chloride 64
ammonium nitrate 136–7
amytal 90
anaesthetics 46, 51, 80, 106
anaesthetists and gas addiction
    106–7
anaphylaxis 34, 38, 39, 41, 42,
    50, 123
Anatomy of Melancholy (Burton)
    6
animals, food additives tested on
    54, 55
Annals of Allergy 25
anthrax 27, 29, 30
antibiotics 5, 31, 80, 93
  in poultry feed 100
  in processed food 102
antibodies 32–3, 41, 42, 61, 143

anti-depressants 24, 68, 94, 149
anti-enzymes 141
antigen 32, 42, 123
antigen/antibody immune
    response 33
antigen/antibody reaction 9,
    38, 39, 60, 143
antihistamine 1, 2, 22, 79, 91,
    94
antioxidants 54, 102
antitoxins 30–31, 34–5
  serum-based 34
antivenin 35
anxiety 7
arsenic, in fish 133
arterio-sclerosis 92
arthritis 120–22
Arthus, Dr Maurice 40
aspirin 41, 42, 79, 123
Assam, deforestation in 19
asthma 15, 23, 27, 40, 121, 162
  and food addiction 102
  caused by allergy 25, 42, 72,
    80–81, 83–4, 142, 144, 146
  Intal for 60
  shot treatment for 39
atmospheric pollution 15
  allergic reaction to xv
atropine 139
attenuation, reduction of
    virulence 30
avoidance manoeuvres 52

bacteria 27, 33, 41
  tuberculosis bacteria 11fn
'balloon bread' 65
bananas 3
barbiturates 80, 90
'barrel effect' 112, 150, 152
Basingstoke District Hospital
    2, 3, 44, 58, 98, 125

behaviour disorders 8, 25, 50, 58, 69, 72, 77, 120, 159
  and food additives 102
  and hydrocarbon inhalation 125
Behring, Emil von 36, 37
benzoyl peroxide 63
Berney, Mrs Pat 50
Binkley, Dr Edward Jr 129–30
biofeedback 155
biscuits 12
Blackley, Dr Charles 23
blackouts 50, 110, 111
Bleuler, Eugen 115
blood serum 40
Borneo, anti-malaria campaign in 18
bowel disorders *see* colitis, colon
brain,
  biochemistry and metabolism of 118–19
  in allergic reactions 6, 50, 119
brain tumour 68
Brave New World (Huxley) 95
bread, white 12, 116
  additives in 57, 63–5
  anti-staling agents in 65
  constituents of 63–5
  fermentation of 64
  softeners 65
breakfast cereals 65
Bridges, Dr Robert 68, 69
British Journal of Psychiatry 118
British Medical Journal 75, 91, 107
British National Oil Corporation 113
British United Provident Association (BUPA) 146
bronchitis 80, *see also* respiratory disorders
bruising 14

bubonic plague 19
Bullock, Dr Thermin 120–22
Burton, Robert 6
butylated hydroxytoluene 54

cabbage 3
cakes 12
calcium, absorption of 65
calcium propionate 63, 65
calcium sulphate 64
Calmette, Dr Albert 35
calories 8, 75, 76
Canadian Arctic Medical Service 77
cancer 5, 49, 107, 119, 120
carbohydrate 8, 9, 75, 76, 77, 119
cardiac problems 44, 45, 50, 124, 143, 162, *see also* heart disease
'Carl', patient 156–7
carrageenan 54
carratoxin 133
Carroll, Dr Murray 120–22
carrot 133
Carson, Rachel 88
cellulose, in processed food 102
central nervous system 7, 77, 91, 125
cereals, refined 10, 12, 20, 103
challenge findings 99, 120, 144, 153, 154
cheese, and allergic illness 65
chemical industry 134, 137
chemical pollution 158
Chemical Victims Club 1, 98, 127, 129, 142
chemically clean environment 6, 78, 125, 164–5
chemicals in air 10, 68, 81, 99
chemicals in food 53–67, 68, 99
chemicals, sensitivity test for 177–8

chemotherapy 31
chicken, battery-reared 98, 99
chicken cholera 30
chicken farming, commercial
　99–101
chlorine 41, 175, 181
chocolate 122
Christmas Carol, A (Dickens) 7
Chronic Disease Center, North
　Carolina 120
cigarette smoke 4, 108, 120, 177
cigarettes 52, 58, 68
citric acid 102
Clarke, Dr John 90
Clean Air Act 15
Cleverdon, Mrs Shirley 4
clinical ecology 10, 12, 16, 22, 23,
　43, 52, 115, 142, 143, 156, 158,
　159
　definition xv
　doctors in the field allergic 49
　literature 25, 44
　society for 23, 25, 39, 123, 156
　units 47, 120, 125, 157
clinical immunology 23
　Department of, Brompton
　Hospital 25
coal tar 174
　in drugs 108, 123
　in processed foods 102, 103,
　112
Coca, Arthur 9, 39
cockroaches 19
coffee 74, 122, 148
cola 122
Coleridge, Samuel Taylor 74
colitis 23, 78, 97, 99, 103, 126,
　146, 163
　in guinea pigs 54
Collison, Dr David 155
colon, irritation of 46, 49

colouring agents in food 12, 56,
　102, 111, 112, 122, 123
common cold 5
convenience foods 54, 67
　additives to 101–3
corn products 9, 122
　in convenience foods 103
cornflour 3
cornstarch, pregelatinized 64
coronary thrombosis 123
cortisone 93
Cousteau, Jacques 134
cowpox 28–9, 30
Crohn's disease 97
Curtis, Michael 74

DDT 88, 136
Daily Mail 5, 112, 158
Dally, Dr Peter 94
Darmady, Dr Judith 122
Darwin, Charles 27
'David', patient 97–8, 101
Delaney, James T. 53
Delaney Hearings 53
dementia praecox *see*
　schizophrenia
dentures, plastic 4
deodorants 4
depression 25, 49, 51, 58, 68, 69,
　72, 74, 75, 77, 78, 97, 98, 105,
　119, 143, 144, 157, 159, 163
dermatitis 101
　peri-oral, rosaceus 93
dermatology 93
desensitization 52, 83, 89, 108,
　143, 151
detergents 113
diagnostic choices 48–9, 146–7
'Diana', patient 69–71, 99, 101
diarrhoea 8, 143
Dickens, Charles 7

diet,
   high fat, high protein, low
      carbohydrate 8–9, 76, 77
   isocaloric 75–6
   rotary diversified 14, 48, 51, 170
   Stone Age 12, 122, 148, 150,
      151, 167–9
dietetic approach 8, 58, 72–3, 78
dinosaurs 18
diphtheria 34, 36
   anti-toxin 36, 37, 40
   bacillus 35, 36
   diphtheria toxin 36
dizziness 8, 44, 109
Doctor's Dilemma, The (Shaw) 33
Doerr, R. 38
Doll, R. and Hill B. A. 120
dopamine levels 118
double-blind tube feeding 58,
   61, 70
drinking water 137
drug addiction 24, 90
drugs 120, 149
   as allergens 37, 42, 95
   additives to 56, 57
   for non-specific symptoms 5, 6,
      13, 21, 46, 49, 73
   psychotropic 69, 94
      anti-allergic properties of 95
   reaction to 121
   safety tests 134
   side effects of 93, 94, 95, 96
   toxicity of 55
Dubois, Rene 141
dust 39, 51, 88, 97
Dutch elm disease 137
dyes,
   FD and C red 57
   in food 54
   in pills and tablets 56–7
dysentery 26

ear, nose and throat symptoms
   13, 14, 39, 142
Eckholm, Eric 18
ecological living space 78
ecology, definition of 26–7
Ecology Party (UK), 138
eggs 10, 24, 72, 77, 99
   in convenience foods 103
Ehrlich, Paul 31–2
Einstein, Albert 158
electro-shock therapy 68, 69
elimination dieting 6, 7, 9, 10, 12,
   see also Stone Age diet
emotional problems 51, 121
environment, adaptability to
   26
Environmental Control Unit,
   Dallas 13, 125
enzymes 119, 141
epilepsy 108, 123, 144
Eskimo, diet of 77
ethanol 108, 180
exclusion diet 126, 148–9, 150,
   157, *see also* Stone Age diet

fainting 1, 2, 3, 4
faith healing 155
fasting treatment 85, *see also*
   elimination dieting, exclusion
   diet, Stone Age diet
fatigue 49, 72, 143, 162
fats 8, 10, 76
   and glucose production 119
   and heart disease 96
feathers 37
Feingold, Dr Ben 123
Finn, Ronald 156
Finor, high-yield wheat 136
'Firemaster' 135
fish 10
   contaminants in 56, 133

Fisons, agricultural chemists 60, 61, 62, 98fn
flavourants in food and drugs 56, 64, 102
Fleming, Sir Alexander 120, 156
floor polish *see* polishes
flour, white 58, 60–62, 63, 64, 97, 98, 127
flour,
  enzyme enriched 63, 64
  flour soya 63, 64
  wholemeal 63
flowers 37
flu-like symptoms 44, 46, 49
fluorocarbon 25, 124
flying doctor service 77
food,
  adulteration of 53–67, 133–4
  hypersensitivity to 122, 123
  labelling of 102
  organic food 140, 149
  organic and commercial distinguished 122
  pollution of 123, 134, 159
  rotation of 131–2, 153
  safety regulations 133
food addiction 24, 162
  masking basis of 85
food additives 6, 12, 14, 20, 51, 72, 97, 102, 108, 149
  animal testing of 54
  as allergens 56
  chronic and sub-acute testing 55
  colouring agents 56, 57
  in chicken farming 100
  LD50 tests 54, 55
  marketing and 65, 66
  natural additives 101–2
  preservatives 20, 56, 65, 66
  processing aids 55, 65, 66
  safety regulations 54–5

statistics on 54
  synthetic additives 101–2
  toxicity studies 54–5, 56, 57
food allergy *see* allergy food
Food and Drugs Administration 53
food contaminants 14, 56, 72, 102
Food, Drug and Cosmetic Act (USA) 53
food families 174–6
food rotation 14, 48, 51, 171
formaldehyde 45, 58, 138, 177, 182
fossil fuels, alternatives to 112
fowl 10
Fowler, Dr John 2
Freedman, Stanley 133
Freud, Sigmund 7, 25, 159
fruits 3, 10, 70, 78, 122, 133
fumes,
  gas *see* gas fumes
  paraffin 79, 108, 124
  petrol *see* motor car exhaust
  printing ink 99
  white spirit 77, 99
  see also anaesthetics, hydrocarbons, petrochemicals
functional disorders 8
fungicidal anti-enzymes 65
fungicides 136
fungus disease in wheat 136–7
fur 37
furniture polish *see* polishes

gas fumes 14, 47fn, 50, 72, 77, 79, 80–81, 104–14, 124, 149
gas gangrene 34
gastro-intestinal disorders 65, 72, 121
geckoe lizards 18–19
general practitioners 69, 97, 145
giddiness 8, 44, 109, 162

glucose 118–19
glue-sniffing 25, 124
glycerides 63, 65
goitre 133
Grose, Peter 157
group therapy 69

Haeckel, Ernst 27
haematuria 125
'hair of the dog' treatment 81–2,
  85, 107
hairspray inhalation 24–5
Hall, Celia 82
Hall, Professor Ross Hume 17
hallucinogens 133
hallucinations 7, 91–2, 115, 125
hangover symptoms 24, 77, 82,
  97, 108, 144
Hansel, Dr French K. 39
hapten 42, 123
Harpers & Queen 6
hay fever 22, 23, 37, 39, 40, 72,
  109, 112, 142, 162
  treatment of 39
Health and Safety Committee of
  Dept of Health 107
heart disease 21, 96, 120, 123
  see also cardiac problems
heart transplants 21
heavy metals 7, 56
Hemmings, William A. 156
high blood pressure 50, 159
Hippocrates 23, 95
Hippocratic tradition 13
Hiroshima 134
histamine 61
hives 37, 40, 41, 122, 123, 142,
  163, *see also* urticaria
homeopathy 155
hormones, in chicken food 100,
  101

Howe, Sir Geoffrey 112–13
Huxley, Aldous 95
hydrocarbons 1, 4, 31
  chlorinated 46, 135, 138
  inhalation of 124–5
hydrogen, radioactive 134
hyperactivity 79, 81, 102, 120, 163
hypersensitivity 142, 143
hypnosis 155
hysteria 81

iatrogenic disease 92–3, 94
ICI 134
idiosyncracy 23, 37, 40, 94, 95,
  96, 143
immunity 26–9, 31, 33, 41, 43
  Ehrlich's side-chain theory of
  32, 41
  shots to boost 51
immunity system, stabilization
  of 60
immunization 31, 34, 159
  active and passive 35, 36
immunology 22, 26, 30, 32, 33,
  41, 143
individual provocative food
  ingestion test 24
individuality, biochemical 95,
  144, *see also* idiosyncracy
indoor air pollution 12, 104–14
industrial accidents 134, 137–8,
  142
industrial effluent 137
influenza 44, 46, 49, 80
  see also flu-like symptoms
inhalant allergy *see* allergy,
  inhalant
infection, infectious disease 22,
  26, 32, 34, 43, 48
  antitoxins against 31
  germ theory of 5, 11fn, 21

insecticides 14, 18–19, 88, 108, 135, 150, 177, 184
  organophosphorus 138–9
instant coffee 68
Intal, for allergic asthma 60–61, 62, 98fn
iodine 133
iron 64
isocaloric diet 75
isocyanate 77
isoflavines 133
itching 57, 72, 163

'James', patient 57–60, 62, 63
Jenner, Edward 27–9, 30
Jeyes fluid 177

Kekwick, Professor Alan 75, 76
Kennedy, President 94
Kenton, Leslie 6
kidney disease 90, 125
Koch, Robert 11
Krantz, J. C. Jr and Carr, C. J. 95

Lancaster General Hospital, Lancaster, Pa. 56
Lancet, 6, 53, 75, 156
Lane, Margaret 100
lard 63
Lawson, Ray 77
L-dopa 92
lead 7, 56
Lentizol 94
leptospirosis 19
levodopa 92
librium 90
lipoxidase 64
liver damage 90, 125
Lockey, Dr Stephen 56, 57, 102, 123

'Loretta', patient 1–3, 126–9
lubricating oil 135–6
Lucretius 23
lungs 104, 142
Lynch, Dr G. Roche 53

McCormick Foods (UK) 133
Macdonald, Dr Betty 75
Mackarness, Dr Richard
  depression 74, 87
  gas allergy of 87
  obesity problem 75–6, 87
  petrochemical allergy 76
  symptoms of 74
  visits Dr Randolph 77–9
McLeave, Hugh 74
McMaster University, Hamilton, Ont. 17
magnesium carbonate 63
malaise 13
malaria, malaria parasite 18, 26
malathion 88
Mandell, Dr Marshall 83
manic depression 7, 118, 126
Marxist myth 119
masked food allergy 24, 97, 144, 145
masking 25, 82, 97, 107
  and unmasking 84–5, 97
  definition 24
  description 82
Massie, Shelagh 4
mast cells 60
measles 26
meat 10, 19, 45, 70, 122
  in convenience foods 103
Mechnikov, Ilya 33
Medinal 90
mental disturbance 7, 72, 90, 92, 95, 118, 119
  see also schizophrenia

mercury 56
Michigan State 135, 138
Michigan, University of 35
Middlesex Hospital, London 75
migraine 37, 65, 78, 121, 143, 157, 162
Milford, Humphrey 74
milk 3, 10, 64, 72, 97, 122, 127
    in convenience foods 103
Miller, Dr Joe 47, 154
Milne, Professor Malcolm 92
mineral oil 56
minerals, in food additives 102
'Miss C. H.', patient 15
Mitchell, Dr, of Montreal 72
Mitchell, Dr Donald 77
Mithridates 35
molasses 3
mono- and di-glycerides 63, 65
monosodium glutamate 102
Montagu, Lady Mary Wortley 28, 29
Morrison, Mrs 127
mortician patient 45, 58
mosquitoes 18
motor car exhaust fumes 1, 3, 41, 47fn, 72, 108
mould 39, 47, 51, 104, 149
mould-retarding agents 65, 102
Mount Sinai Hospital, NY 135
'Mrs A.', patient 13–14
'Mrs D.', patient 109–12
'Mrs K.P.', patient 79–81
mycotoxins 136
Myers, Norman 19
myristicin 133

Nalcrom (Intal) 62, 98, 154
National Health Service 68–9, 146, 147
natural therapy 155

nerve gases 138–9, 140
nervous tension 24
neuritis 136
neurosis 11
neurotransmitters 118
News Chronicle 74, 75, 82
niacin 64
nickel 41
nitrogen levels in water 137
Noon, Leonard 39
nor-adrenalin levels 118
Not All in the Mind (Mackarness) 116
nuclear power programmes 134
nucleotides 102
Nursing Times 154

obesity 8, 9, 74, 75, 76, 77, 157, 159
oedema 70
ointments, steroid 93
organic feeding 70–71
orthomolecular treatment 154–5
osteopathy 155

painkillers 80
paint solvents 76–7, 108, 124, 150
Panton, Louis 158
paraffin fumes 79, 108, 124
parasympathetic nerves 139–40
Park Prewett Hospital 69
Parkinsonism 92
passive immunity 34, 35, 36
Pasteur, Louis 27, 29, 31, 35, 140fn
Pasteur Institute, Paris 35
patients cited
    'Carl' 156–7
    'David' 97–8, 101
    'Diana' 69–71, 99, 101
    'James' 57–60, 62, 63

patients cited, *continued*
  'Miss C.H.' 15
  mortician 45, 58
  'Mrs A.' 13–14
  'Mrs D.' 109–12
  'Mrs K.P.' 79–81
  'Patrick' 122–3
  'Pauline' 82–3
  Phipps, James 28
  'Sharon' 24–5
'Patrick', patient 122–3
Paul, Dr David 124
'Pauline', patient 82–3
Pawan, Dr Gaston 75, 76, 156
peanut 122, 148, 174
  in convenience food 103
penicillin 31, 120
peptic ulcer syndrome 8, 163
Pepys, Professor Jack 25, 156
perfumes 181
pesticides 12, 78, 89, 100, 140
  residues in food 54
petrochemicals 4, 14, 51, 76, 98,
    107, 119, 140, 165
  for desensitization 84
  in aerosols 25, 124
  in processed food 102, 103
  'nature's' 47fn
phagocytosis 33
phenobarbitol 57, 110
phenol 84, 175, 181–2
Phipps, James 28
phlebitis 44
Piriton 1
Pirquet, Clemens von 22, 38, 40
pituitary hormones 84
plastic, as allergen 46, 50–51, 150
Police Surgeons' Association 90
polishes 4, 98, 125, 127, 128, 149
pollen 22, 23, 39, 47, 51, 60–61,
    88, 97, 109, 149

pollutants 7, 71
polychlorinated biphenyl (PCB)
  135–6, 138, 139
Portier, Paul 38
Portuguese man-of-war 37
potassium bromate 63, 64
pregnancy 126–9, 130, 131
preservatives 12, 20, 56, 65, 102
Private Patients Plan (PPP) 146
procain 80
prophylaxis 34, 37, 38, 83
protein 8
  in convenience foods 101
  in diet 76, 119
  serum proteins 41, 42, 123
protein molecule 31–2
psychiatrists 11, 25
  physicians' distrust of 2
psychiatry 7, 50
  and schizophrenia 118
psychological disturbance 49,
  146
psychology 7
psychosis 125, 126
psychosomatic disorders 7, 8, 11,
  26, 120
  treatment of 12
Pugh, Dr 127
pupil enlargement 118

Queen Charlotte's Hospital for
  Women, London 119
Queen Elizabeth Hospital,
  Birmingham 107

rabies 30
  vaccination against 34, 38
radishes 133
Raffle, Dr Andrew 91
ragweed hay fever 39

Randolph, Dr Théron G. 44, 46, 49, 71–4, 77, 87–8, 109, 110, 111, 156, 157
  and chemical allergy 12, 25, 72, 81, 105
  and specific adaptation syndrome 85
  and toxicologists 56
  BBC interview with 72–3
  fasting procedure 6, 9, 10, 73
  on gas-induced depression 105–6
  on indoor air pollution 108, 111
  on synthetic food additives 102, 111, 123
Randolph, Mrs 78
rats 19
Rea, Professor William xv, 13, 15, 43–9, 51, 58, 107, 123, 125, 156
  'barrel effect' 112, 150, 152
  dieting procedure 45, 48
Rea, Mrs Vera 43, 46, 49
Reader's Digest 96
reductional research 118, 120, 143
Reilly, Dr William 91
respiratory disorders 13, 15, 25, 44–5, 79–80, 104, 116, 142
rheumatic pains 72, 78, 81, 143
rheumatism 120–22
riboflavin 64
Richet, Professor Charles 37–8, 39, 40, 42
Rinkel, Dr Herbert J. 9, 23, 24–5, 39, 44, 85
road accidents 90
Roux, Dr Pierre 35, 36
Rowe, Dr Albert 9, 23, 24, 39, 44, 72
Royal Society 28
Ryvita 3

St Mary's Hospital, Paddington 39, 156
salt, common 55, 63, 64, 102
Salvarsan 31
Samman, Dr Peter 93
Sandler, Dr Morton 119
sardines 3
scarlet fever 80
Schaudin, F. 120
Schick, Dr Bela 40
schizophrenia 7, 115–16, 118, 119, 126, 157
  biological-experimental approach to 118
sea-anemone 37–8
sedatives 80, 90–91
Selikoff, Professor Irving 135
Selye, Professor Hans 84
sensitivity, individual 88–9, 98
serum proteins 41, 42
serum sickness 37, 40
Sewall, Dr Henry 34–5
'Sharon', patient 24–5
Shaw, George Bernard 33
shock 41
side-chain theory of immunity 32, 41
Silent Spring (Carson) 88
Simmons, Lieutenant George 92
skim milk powder 63, 64
skin rash 1, 2, 14, 72, 80, 142, 162, 163
  see also hives, urticaria
skin tests 9, 39, 47, 49
sleeping sickness 31, 33
smallpox 27–30, 36
  vaccination against 33, 38
smells 113–14
smoking 52, 98, 128, 149–50
snake venom 34–5
sodium cromoglycate 60, 62, 154

soft drinks 12, 122
solvent inhalation and addiction 124–5
soya flour 61, 63, 103
specific adaptation syndrome 85, 157, 158, 159
specific maladaptation 144
spreading phenomenon 15
spring water 3, 6, 10, 14
starch, processed 12
  in convenience foods 101
steroids 15, 22, 93, 94, 97, 98
stilboestrol 101
Stone Age diet 12, 122, 148, 167–9
stress 84
sugar 3, 12, 63, 82–3, 122, 127
  in convenience foods 101
suicide attempts, drugs used in 94
sulphonamides 80
Sunday Telegraph 100
surgery 13, 21
sweating 21, 162
Swedish Covenant Hospital, Chicago 6, 9, 78
sweeteners, in convenience foods 102, 103
sweets 12
  additives in 54
syphylis 31, 120

2–4.D (2–4 dichlorophenoxy-acetic acid) 136
tartrazine 123
Taylor, G. S. and Hern, W. S. 124
tea 103, 122
terpenes 47, 51, 107
tetanus 34
tetracycline 93
thalidomide 134
Thames Water Authority 137
thiamine mononitrate 64

Three Mile Island atomic power station, Pa. 134
tobacco 52, 98, 113, 119
Today magazine 82, 93
Todd, Susan 82–3, 154
toluene 77
Tomlin, P. J. 107
toxic poisoning 7
toxicity studies 54–5
  chronic and sub-acute testing 55
toxins 37
trace mineral deficiency 7, 129
tranquillizers 24, 58, 90, 94, 149, 175
travel phobia 8
tricalcium phosphate 63
Trypanosoma gambiense 31
Tryptizol 94
tsetse fly 31
tuberculosis 26, 68
  bacterium 11fn
  vaccination against 30
turpentine 99
typhoid fever 32–3
  vaccine against 30, 33

UK Committee on Safety of Medicines 134
urticaria 1, 2, 3, 4, 37, 40, 41, 57, 122, 142, 162, 163
  and food additives 102, 123
  treatment of 39

vaccination, vaccines 22, 29
  cholera 30, 34
  diphtheria 30
  rabies 34, 38
  smallpox 30, 33, 34, 38
  tuberculosis 30
  typhoid 30, 33, 34
valium 90

variolation 28, 29
vasculitis 44, 162
Vaughan, Dr Victor 41
Vaughan, Warren T. 39
vegetables 10, 70, 78, 122, 133
venereal disease 119, 120
Virchous, Rudolph 156
vitamin B 64
  synthetic 80, 103
vitamins, added 102
vomiting 8, 80

water xiii, 137
weed spraying 136
weight loss 80, 111
Westminster Hospital, London
  92–3, 94
wheat, fungus disease on 136
wheat products 9, 72, 103,
  116–18, 122, 172

white cells 33
white spirit 77, 99
whooping cough 26
William, Dr Roger J. 95
Wilson, Professor Cedric 156
Windscale 134
withdrawal symptoms 24, 158
Woman's Journal 82
Woman's Own 4
Worldwatch Institute 18
Worthing Gazette 50
Wright, Sir Almroth 156
Wright-Fleming Institute 156

xylene 77

yeast 58, 60, 63, 64
  in convenience foods 103
'yeast food' 64

Vernon Coleman
Stress Control £1.25

Stress is the one constant factor besieging almost every individual in our overcrowded, pressured and city-focused world. It causes depression and sleepless nights, family tensions, sexual difficulties, illnesses of every kind.

Vernon Coleman, an experienced family doctor and writer on many medical topics, explains how controlling stress can be the way to a happier and healthier life.

medical editor-in-chief: Dr Eric J. Trimmer
The Visual Dictionary of Sex £5.95

With more than 400 illustrations, many in full colour, *The Visual Dictionary of Sex* is an authoritative, frank and practical guide to every aspect of human sexual life.

In one book, here is everything anyone could ever want to know about sex and sexuality.

edited by Sigmund Stephen Miller
Symptoms
the complete home medical encyclopedia £2.50

The new medical encyclopedia — accurate, comprehensive, easy to use, sensible — enabling the reader to track down any symptom of ill health and identify, quickly and accurately, the causal disorder. *Symptoms* will tell you exactly what is wrong, and guide you in what action to take, whether a simple home remedy, or whether to seek advice from your doctor. Each section of the book is written by a specialist in one area of the body, and there is also a glossary of medical terms, comprehensive cross-indexes, and a guide to maintaining a high standard of general good health.

David Lewis
The Secret Language of Your Child £1.50

Children can communicate before they have learned to speak. This fascinating book tells how they use this 'secret language' and what it means.

'A language of looks and gestures that can be even more eloquent than the most fluent speech' TIMES EDUCATIONAL SUPPLEMENT

'A book with a serious and important purpose ... an excellent book and, what is more, fun' PSYCHOLOGY TODAY

Lauren Elder
with Shirley Streshinsky
And I Alone Survived 90p

Not since *Alive!* has there been a survival story like this one.

Lauren Elder set out in a light aircraft with the pilot and his girlfriend on a joyride, skyborne sightseeing over the splendour of the Sierra Nevada range. When the plane hit the mountain, the joyride turned into a nightmare. After a night of sub-zero temperatures, Laura, the only survivor, faced a fearsome 8000-foot climb down to safety ...

'Vividly recreates a nightmare ordeal' YORKSHIRE POST

Sheila Hailey
I Married a Best Seller 95p

Arthur Hailey is the author of *Airport, Hotel, Overload* ... and a whole string of blockbusting world bestsellers. Sheila Hailey is his wife. Her story is one of ups and downs, of being immensely wealthy and of scraping together small change for the price of a cinema ticket. It is a story of love and life and staying married ... without doubt one of the most candid, caution-to-the-winds life stories anybody's ever put on paper.

'A determinedly honest character study ... a murderous but endearing assault on the private files of a marriage sanctuary' DAILY MAIL

Michael Pearson
Tears of Glory
the betrayal of Vercours £1.25

The Vercours Massif, 1944 : two days after the Normandy landings this vast natural fortress was the scene of the most tragic action in the bloodstained annals of the French Resistance. The Tricolor fluttered briefly over the Frenchmen who had flocked to the Maquis in the face of twenty thousand German troops. The promised Allied air support on which their success depended never arrived — Vercours was betrayed, and the outcome was inevitable.

'An enthralling though tragic narrative . . . crystal-clear description of tactics, fighting and terrain' DAILY TELEGRAPH

edited and introduced by Hugh Trevor-Roper
The Goebbels Diaries: the last days £1.95

'His great gestures were hymns of hate. His chosen form of action was destructive violence . . .' *Hugh Trevor-Roper*

'A daemonic master of words . . . Goebbels' diaries make absorbing reading' DAILY TELEGRAPH

'This volume presents the material surviving from the period between February 27 and April 9 1945 — the period of the collapse of the Third Reich. Goebbels' diaries from the bunker are a hot line from *two seconds to midnight*' GUARDIAN

Robert Taylor
The Fifth Estate £1.95

Are Britain's unions too weak or too powerful ? Robber barons or failed agents of social justice ? Are they responsible for Britain's postwar economic decline, or a constructive force ?

Labour correspondent of the *Observer*, Robert Taylor examines such questions, giving a highly readable profile of the trade union movement, its history and structure. Revised and updated to the May 1979 General Election, this will become the classic analysis of the British unions in the late twentieth century.

'Invaluable . . . entertaining, informative and accurate' ECONOMIST

'Essential reading' SCOTSMAN

Christopher Timothy
Vet Behind the Ears 80p

TV's 'James Herriot' tells his own story, as entertaining, touching and truly hilarious as James Herriot's stories themselves – the splendid books of a vet's life in the Yorkshire Dales which have sold in millions across the globe, and which, when made into a TV series, brought relief from imminent unemployment to Christopher Timothy, and went on to become a hit on the small screen, making him a household name.

James Herriot
All Things Wise and Wonderful £1.75
the third Herriot omnibus edition

The third Herriot omnibus takes up the story of the world's favourite vet at the outbreak of World War Two – swapping gumboots for goggles, he's transported from the Darrowby dales to an RAF training camp somewhere in England. Bashing the square or up in the air, he's daydreaming of the life – and the livestock – he left behind ...

'Provokes a chuckle, or a lump in your throat, in every chapter' DAILY MIRROR